Peripheral Musculoskeletal
Ultrasound Atlas

Peripheral Musculoskeletal Ultrasound Atlas

S. Marcelis, B. Daenen
and M.A. Ferrara

Edited by R.F. Dondelinger

750 illustrations

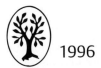 1996

Georg Thieme Verlag
Stuttgart · New York

Thieme Medical Publishers, Inc.
New York

Robert F. Dondelinger, M. D.
Professor and Chairman

S. Marcelis, M. D.

B. Daenen, M. D.

M. A. Ferrara, M. D.

University Hospital Sart Tilman
University of Liège
B 35
B-4000 Liège
Belgium

Library of Congress Cataloging-in-Publication Data

Peripheral musculoskeletal ultrasound atlas / edited by
R. F. Dondelinger: in collaboration with S. Marcelis,
B. Daenen, and M. A. Ferrara.
p. cm.
Includes bibliographical references and index.
ISBN 3-13-102771-1 (GTV). – ISBN 0-86577-592-3 (TMP)
1. Musculoskeletal system – Ultrasonic imaging – Atlases.
I. Dondelinger, R. F.
[DNLM: 1. Musculoskeletal Diseases – ultrasonography –
atlases.
2. Extremities – ultrasonography – atlases. WE 17 P442
1996]
RC925.7.P46 1996
616.7'07543 – dc20
DNLM/DLC
for Library of Congress   95-39513
          CIP

Cover drawing by Renate Stockinger

© 1996 Georg Thieme Verlag, Rüdigerstraße 14,
D-70469 Stuttgart, Germany
Thieme Medical Publishers, Inc., 381 Park Avenue South,
New York, N.Y. 10016

Typesetting by Druckhaus Götz GmbH,
D-71636 Ludwigsburg
(CCS-Textline [Linotronic 630])
Printed in Germany by K. Grammlich GmbH, Pliezhausen

ISBN 3-13-102771-1 (GTV, Stuttgart)
ISBN 0-86577-592-3 (TMP, New York)   2 3 4 5 6

Preface

In 1975, a distinguished professor of radiology stated that "all ultrasound is artifact." He was probably correct at that time, but we have advanced far since then. Ultrasound examination has been proven to reflect detailed anatomy with confidence in almost all locations from fetal to adult age. The ultrasound beam, focused in various geometries, can be applied transcutaneously or with endoscopic approaches in the human body. Therefore, it is surprising that the peripheral musculoskeletal system has not yet attracted the attention that is deserves. In fact, the number of textbooks remains scarce compared to those devoted to musculoskeletal MRI, and despite the many scientific papers that have been published, clinical application of ultrasound to the musculoskeletal system still remains limited in many Departments of Radiology. Constant progress in MRI, which is able to exquisitely depict the bone marrow and the surrounding soft tissues, favored extensive investigation in various pathologies of the locomotor system, capturing most of the attention and thus diminishing the interest in less prestigious imaging modalities such as ultrasound.

However, state-of-the-art high-resolution ultrasound equipment has made it possible to accurately image most disease processes or injuries, involving even the smallest structures. When applied on an emergency basis, diagnoses such as muscular or tendon tears, hematomas, fractures, joint effusions, foreign bodies, and others are confirmed within a few minutes. These findings would have escaped conventional radiology, and MRI is not immediately available most of the time.

Ultrasound is versatile, quick, and places the radiologist in close contact with the patient, thus enhancing full integration of imaging and clinical findings. During the writing process of the manuscript and captions of the illustrations of this atlas, I was impressed by the number and the variety of pathological cases that Dr. Stefaan Marcelis was able to collect in only a short period of time. This proved, to a sufficient extent, the clinical usefulness of the technique. It also became clear that an extensive knowledge of detailed musculoskeletal anatomy is required, involving structures that are usually overlooked on other imaging modalities. Furthermore, a thorough understanding of ultrasound examination techniques and of pathophysiology and pathology of the diseases is absolutely mandatory. There is no doubt that it takes many months of full-time training to become an expert in musculoskeletal ultrasound. Radiologists who are already familiar with 3-D representation and who have access to the other imaging techniques are in the best position to judge the strengths and limits of all techniques.

The present atlas should stimulate radiologists in training, radiologists, and other specialists dealing with the pathologies of the musculoskeletal system to learn more about ultrasound examination and to help them with the recognition of elementary signs and pathological entities. This will thus enable them to formulate quick and definite answers to many clinical questions.

Liège, Spring 1996

Robert F. Dondelinger, M.D.
Professor and Chairman

Acknowledgements

We want to offer special thanks to Karine Lambert, M.D., from the Department of Medical Imaging at the University Hospital of Liège, who graciously offered her help in completing several chapters. We are also grateful to Paul Beeckman, M.D., from the Department of Radiology at Sint Andries Ziekenhuis of Tielt, for the collection of interesting cases and express our thanks to the colleagues of the Department of Orthopaedic Surgery and Physical Medicine of Sint Andries Ziekenhuis of Tielt. Special acknowledgements go to Roger Lemaire, M.D., Professor and Chairman of the Department of Orthopaedic Surgery, Jean-Michel Crielaard, M.D., Professor and Chairman of the Department of Physical Medicine, and to Michel Malaise, M.D., Chief of the Department of Rheumatology, for continuous cooperation between their teams and the Department of Medical Imaging at the University Hospital of Liège.

We recognize the meticulous artwork of Pierre Paquet, who produced the illustrations, and the commitment of Anne Piron, who typed the manuscript. Finally, we acknowledge the unrestricted support from all of the members of Georg Thieme Verlag who made this publication possible.

Table of Contents

General Part 1

Equipment 2

Examination Technique 3

Artifacts 6
Shadow 6
Absent Shadow: Beamwidth Artifact 6
Enhancement by Transmission 7
Anisotropy 8
Refractile Shadowing 9
Reverberation 10

Normal Appearances 11
Muscle 11
Tendon 12
Ligament 13
Periosteum and Bone 14
Joint Capsule, Bursa, and Synovium 15
Hyaline Cartilage 16
Fibrocartilage 16
Vessel 17
Nerve 18
Fat and Skin 19

Basic Signs of Pathology 20
Muscle 20
   Hypertrophy and Atrophy 20
   Elongation and Partial Rupture 21
   Complete Rupture 22
   Hematoma 22
   Crush Injury 23
   Delayed-Onset Muscle Soreness 23
   Healing 24
   Healing Complications 25
   Myositis Ossificans 26
   Compartment Syndrome 27
   Accessory Muscle 28
   Herniation 29
Tendon 30
   Acute Tendinitis 30
   Chronic Tendinitis 31

   Tendinitis, Miscellaneous 32
   Partial Rupture 33
   Complete Rupture 34
Ligament 35
   Injury 35
Bursa 36
   Acute Bursitis 36
   Chronic Bursitis 36
   Inflammatory and Infectious Bursitis 37
   Hemorrhagic Bursitis 38
   Metabolic Bursitis 38
Capsule 39
   Effusion 39
   Septic Effusion 40
   Loose bodies 40
   Synovial Thickening 41
Cartilage 42
   Traumatic 42
   Degenerative 42
Arteries 43
   Pathology 43
Veins 44
   Pathology 44
Nerve 45
   Inflammation 45
   Neurinoma and Neurofibroma 46
Cortex and Periosteum 47
   Fracture 47
   Stress Fracture 48
   Osteomyelitis 49
Evaluation of Orthopaedic Procedures 50
   Callus Formation 50
   Infection 50
   Prostheses 51
Skin 52
   Scar 52
   Edema 53
   Lipoma 54
   Cyst 55
Foreign Body 56

Puncture 58

Normal and Pathologic Regional Ultrasound: Upper Extremities 59

Shoulder 60
Anatomy 60
Pathology 65
   Rotator Cuff : Full-Thickness Tear 65
   Rotator Cuff : Partial-Thickness-
   and Intrasubstance Tears 68
   Impingement Syndrome 69
   Calcified Tendinitis 71

Biceps Tendinitis 72
Biceps Tendon Rupture 73
Biceps Tendon Luxation 73
Effusion 74
Milwaukee Shoulder 75
Traumatic Injury 76

Table of Contents

Upper Arm 77
Anatomy 77

Elbow 79
Anatomy 79
Pathology 84
   Effusion and Loose Bodies 84
   Olecranon Bursitis 85
   Lateral Epicondylitis 86
   Biceps and Triceps Tendon Pathology 87
   Ulnar Nerve Entrapment 88
   Rheumatoid Arthritis 89

Forearm 90
Anatomy 91

Wrist 92
Anatomy 92
Pathology 97
   Arthrosynovial Cyst 97
   Ganglion Cyst 98

Carpe Bossu 99
Scaphoid Fracture 99
Gout 100
De Quervain's Tenosynovitis 101
Tendinitis and Tenosynovitis 102
Rheumatoid Arthritis 103
Guyon's Canal Syndrome 104
Carpal Tunnel Syndrome 104
Triangular Fibrocartilage Tear 105
Amyloidosis 106

Hand 107
Anatomy 107
Pathology 111
   Tenosynovitis 111
   Rheumatoid Arthritis 112
   Tendon Rupture 113
   Osteoarthritis 114
   Dupuytren's Contracture 114
   Tenosynovial Cyst 115
   Gamekeeper's Thumb 116

Normal and Pathologic Regional Ultrasound: Lower Extremities 117

Infant Hip 118
Anatomy 118

Hip 121
Anatomy 121
Pathology 126
   Effusion 126
   Effusions in Children 127
   Bursitis 128
   Tendinitis 129
   Sports Injuries 130
   Hamstring Tendinitis 131

Thigh 132
Anatomy 132

Knee 135
Anatomy 135
Pathology 140
   Effusion 140
   Baker's Cyst 141
   Popliteal Masses 142
   Tendinitis 143
   Patellar Tendinitis 144
   Osgood – Schlatter Disease 145
   Quadriceps Tendon Rupture and Tendinitis . 146
   Pes Anserinus Tendinitis 147
   Retinaculum/Synovial Impingement 147
   Bursitis 148
   Medial Collateral Ligament Injury 149
   Lateral Collateral Ligament Injury 150

Shin Splint 150
Cruciate Ligament Injury 151
Meniscal Tear and Cyst 152
Ganglion Cyst 153
Periosteal Desmoid 154

Leg 155
Anatomy 155

Ankle 157
Anatomy 157
Pathology 162
   Effusions and Loose Body 162
   Achilles Tendon Tendinitis 163
   Achilles Tendon Rupture 165
   Peroneal Tenosynovitis 167
   Peroneal Tendon Luxation 168
   Peroneal Tendon Rupture 168
   Posterior Tibial Tendon Tenosynovitis 169
   Posterior Tibial Tendon Rupture 170
   Bursitis 171
   Ligament Injury 172
   Accessory Soleus Muscle 173
   Haglund Deformity 174
   Cystic Masses 175

Foot 176
Anatomy 176
Pathology 181
   Rheumatoid Arthritis 181
   Gout 182

Table of Contents

Cystic Mass 183

Bone Injury 184

Plantar Fasciitis 185

Ledderhose Disease 186

Morton Neuroma 187

References 189

Index 199

Introduction

The purpose of this atlas is to give an overview of the most common applications of high-definition ultrasound in the field of musculoskeletal pathology. The majority of the images were obtained with a commercially available 7.5 MHz probe on Performa (acoustic imaging) equipment, manufactured by Dornier Medizintechnik GmbH.

Studies realized on an experimental basis, such as 3-D images or examinations with a 15 or 20 MHz probe, are deliberately excluded in this overview, but can provide additional information in specific settings.

The systematic approach and the anatomy of the different joints of the upper and lower limb are illustrated. Representative ultrasound scans of the inter-articular regions complete the anatomic illustrations. The ultrasound evaluation of thoracic and abdominal wall and head and neck region is excluded. Examination techniques, pitfalls, and artifacts are explained and demonstrated. Ultrasound signs of regional and basic pathologic entities are discussed and illustrated with typical examples.

Only common benign tumors with typical ultrasound features are described. The ultrasound features of the dysplastic hip are only briefly summarized, since they have been extensively described in the literature. The interested reader will find these references included in the subject-oriented bibliography. A 1 cm distance is indicated on each images, serving as a reference for its magnification.

General Part

Equipment

Examination Technique

Artifacts

Normal Appearances

Basic Signs of Pathology

Puncture

Equipment

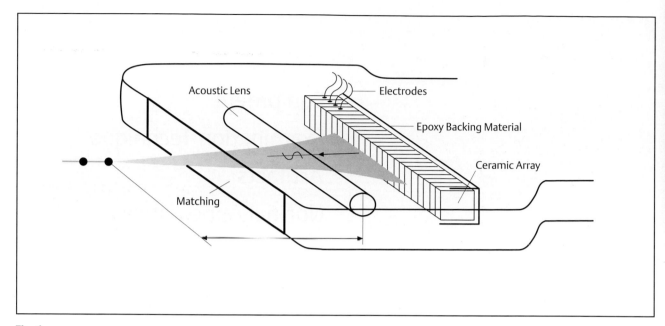

Fig. 1
Schematic representation of basic components of an ultrasound transducer.

Sound is reflected at the interfaces of materials with different acoustic impedance. The angle of incidence should be 90° to the structures evaluated in order to keep refraction to a minimum and to ensure maximum reflection. The degree of absorption of a sound beam is directly proportional to its frequency. The transmitting and receiving electronics have improved in recent years. The array's bandwidth characteristics have been optimized, while sidelobe artifacts at different depths have been suppressed. The receiver electronics must have an extremely large dynamic range and bandwidth to preserve all the subtle differences in amplitude between the received echoes. Only then a high contrast resolution, i.e., the ability to differentiate subtle tissue densities and variations in structure and a high spatial resolution, as well as the ability to distinguish small structures, can be guaranteed. This is now obtained by a dual dynamic delay technique.

Parallel programming of the delays allows one delay module to operate during the time the unused module is programmed to a new focusing zone. A summing architecture fits all the information together free of noise. Systems that have poor dynamic range performance because of noise mask very low-level signals and lose information. A limitation in the system's ability to handle large signals tends to overload on large signals and will also lose information. Thus, not only the number of elements inside a transducer, but rather the way these elements are excited in time will determine the resolution of the ultrasound image. By allowing the user to select multiple focusing zones, lateral and axial resolution can be optimized.

Using a ceramic polymer composite material for the array and epoxy backing material minimizes the loss of acoustic energy during transmission and reception. The images in this book were obtained with a 7.5 MHz linear scan-head, a 5 MHz convex array transducer, and a 5 MHz linear array transducer. A few images were obtained with a 10 MHz linear array transducer.

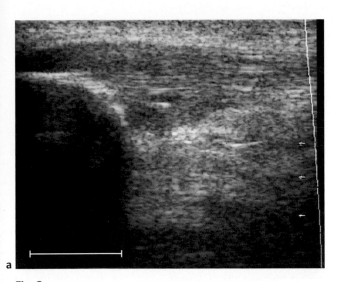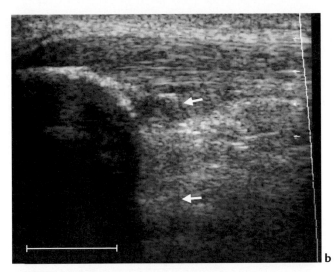

Fig. 2
Scan before correct focusing (**a**). After appropriate focusing, the image becomes sharper and a calcification with acoustic shadow (→) becomes evident in this patient with chronic fissuring tendinitis at the proximal pole of the patellar tendon (jumper's knee) (**b**).

High-quality linear array probes of high frequency are used to evaluate superficial structures. Correct present and gain should be looked for. Appropriate focusing is vital. The study should be directed in various planes and in a comparative way.

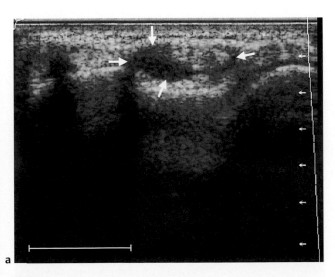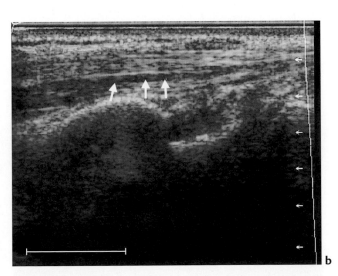

Fig. 3
The amount of fluid surrounding the extensor digitorum tendon in this patient is better evaluated in a transverse scan (→) (**a**) than in a longitudinal plane (**b**).

Examination Technique

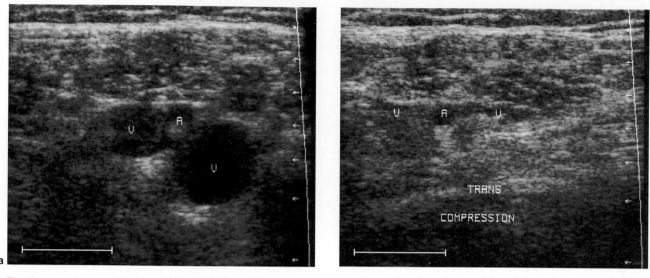

Fig. 4
The normal posterior tibial veins are anechoic dilated structures (**a**) that are compressible (**b**), proving their patency.

In contrast to other imaging modalities, ultrasound offers a unique opportunity to evaluate the soft tissue structures in a perpendicular or parallel plane, even when they have an oblique or curved direction. Compression can provide important information: it proves venous patency, evaluates the synovial thickness, and provides information on tenderness.

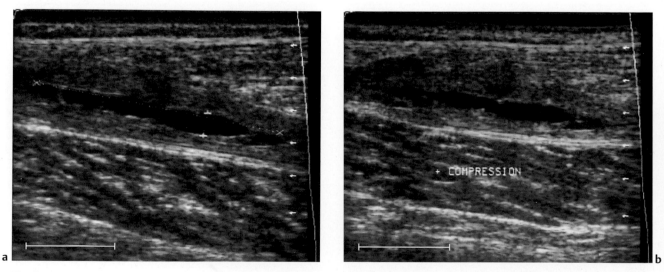

Fig. 5
A small elongated muscle rupture can mimic a deep vein (**a**) but is not compressible (**b**).

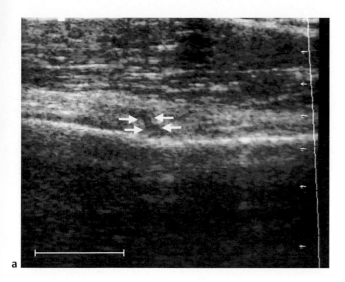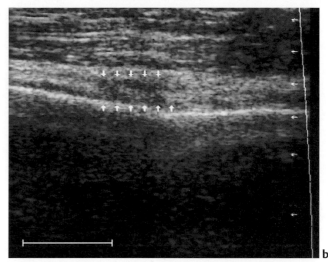

Fig. 6
Complete rupture of the biceps tendon in a longitudinal plane (**a**) becomes more evident with contraction (→) (**b**).

Contraction or strain can be used routinely to detect or evaluate musculotendinous or ligamentous lesions.

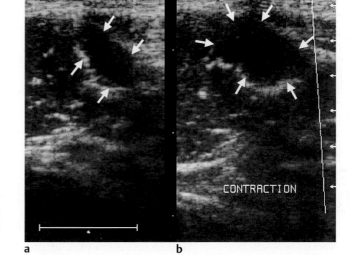

Fig. 7
On a transverse scan, the gap in this partial muscle rupture (**a**) becomes larger on contraction, so that the extent of the lesion is more easily seen (**b**).

Artifacts

Shadow

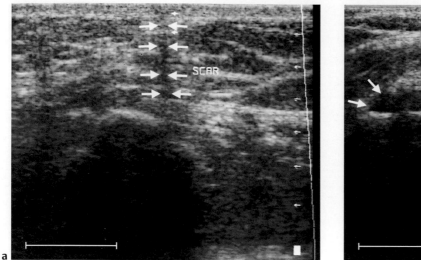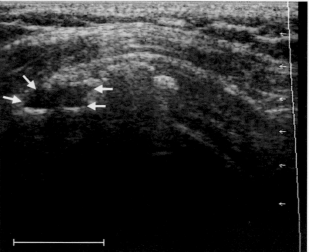

Fig. 8
A cutaneous scar causes an acoustic shadow (→) (**a**). Calcifications in the rotator cuff induce shadows (→) and can mimic tendinous tears (**b**).

A shadow corresponds to a signal void, and can be induced by scar tissue or normal fibrous septa as present in muscle or subcutaneous fat, or by calcifications or bony surfaces.

Absent Shadow : Beamwidth Artifact

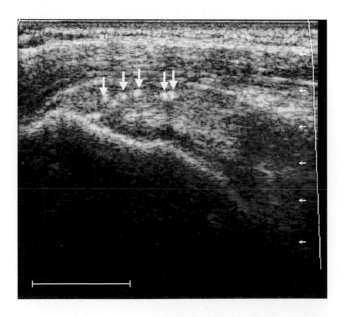

Fig. 9
Multiple hyperechoic spots (→) are seen in the insertion of the supraspinatus tendon; the smallest calcifications do not cause a shadow.

If calcifications are too small in relation to the beamwidth, no shadow will be present.

Enhancement by Transmission

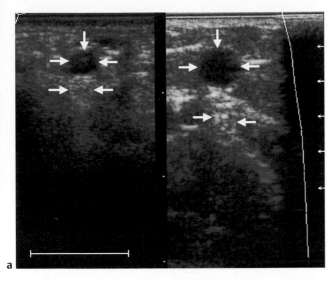
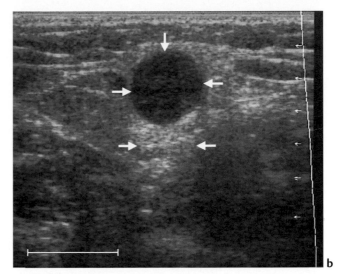

Fig. 10
A posterior enhancement is seen at the level of the radial artery and basilic vein (→) in a transverse scan (**a**). Enhancement by transmission is seen posterior to this hematoma (→) (**b**).

The time gain compensation produces an amplification of the echoes from deeper structures in an exponential way in relation to the echo time. This explains the increased echogenicity of tissues in a location deep to structures that have a relatively low ultrasound attenuation. This observation can be made in normal anatomic structures such as vessels, or in pathologic conditions such as cysts or inflamed tendons.

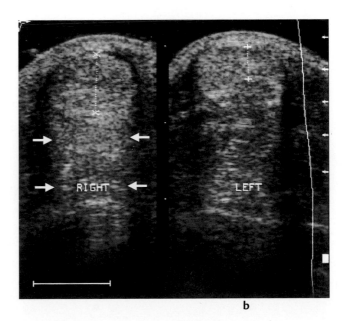

Fig. 11
An acute tendinitis of the Achilles tendon on the right side markedly enhances the posterior fat (→) (**a**) in comparison to the normal left side (**b**).

Artifacts

Anisotropy

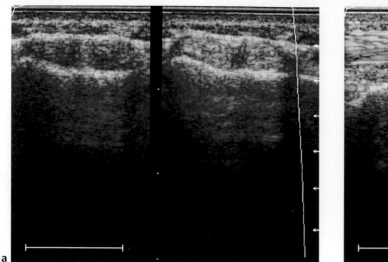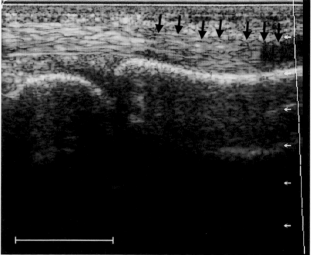

Fig. 12
The tendons at the anterior radial border change their echogenicity when the transducer is angled (**a**). The echogenicity of the flexor indicis tendon decreases in its curved course on the proximal phalanx (→) (**b**).

Muscles and tendons can vary their echogenicity when examined at different angles. Correct evaluation necessitates a strict perpendicular approach.

This peculiar property can be helpful to differentiate tendons from a hyperechoic surrounding tissue (e.g., tendons at the wrist).

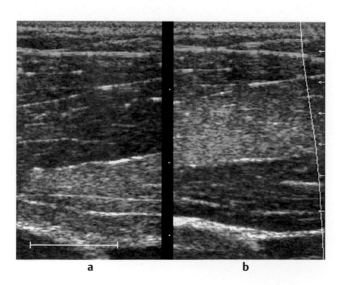

Fig. 13
Changing echogenicity of the radial extensor muscles is obtained by varying the examination angle.

Refractile Shadowing

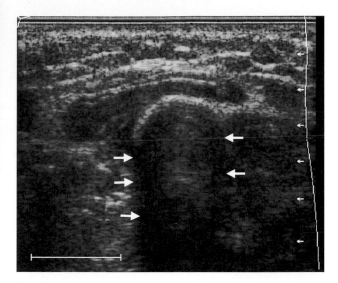

Fig. 14
Refractile shadows are seen at both margins of a curved cortex (→).

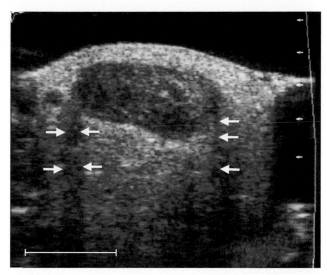

Fig. 15
Refractile shadows in Achilles tendinitis (→).

No echoes are returned at the lateral margins of a highly curved surface. This phenomenon is also called critical angle shadowing, and can be seen in normal and pathologic conditions.

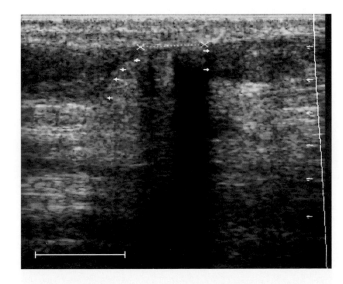

Fig. 16
In Achilles tendon rupture, refractile shadows are seen at the free tendon ends (→) and invaginating fat.

Artifacts

Reverberation

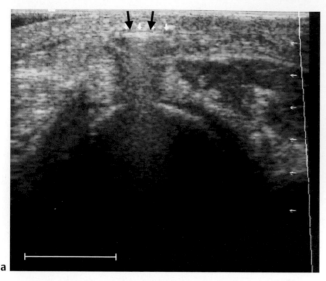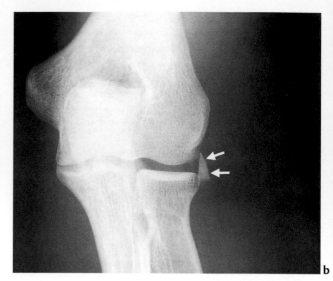

Fig. 17
A comet's-tail artifact is seen in the soft tissues of the elbow due to a glass fragment (→) (**a**), also visible on the radiograph (→) (**b**).

Reverberation artifacts are caused by metallic or glass objects. The repetitive echoic bands found at intervals equal to the object's thickness diminish with distance from the object and create a comet's tail appearance. This comet's-tail artifact crosses tissue boundaries. Air also produces reverberation artifacts, giving a posterior shadow that contains echoes, the so-called dirty shadow.

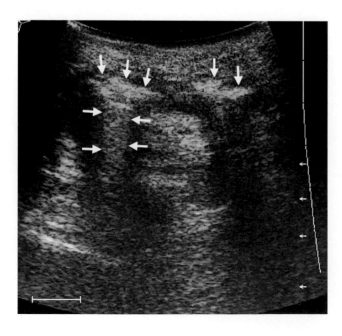

Fig. 18
Air bubbles in a collection of an infected hip prosthesis give dirty shadows that contain reverberation echoes (→).

Muscle

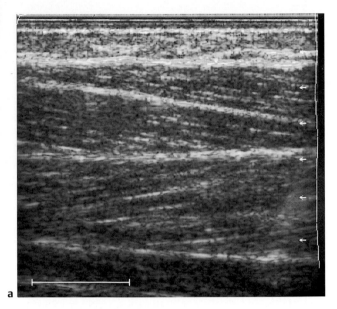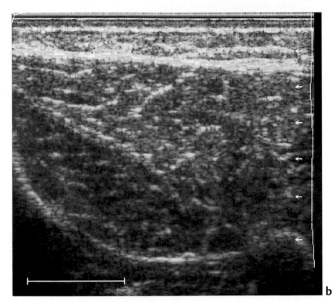

Fig. 19
Longitudinal scan (**a**).Transverse scan (**b**).

The sonographic appearance of normal skeletal muscle in a longitudinal section is composed of homogeneous, multiple, fine, parallel echoes. These parallel echoic striae are generated by the connective tissue that surrounds the bundles of fibers or perimysium and project over a hypoechoic background, representing the bulk of the muscle fibers. The fibers have a parallel course toward a central or a peripheral aponeurosis, ending in a tendon distally. On transverse scans, the cross-sectional perimysium appears as scattered dot echoes. This feathery appearance is due to multiple muscle fasciculi surrounded by fibroadipose septae or perimysium. A brightly echoic outer margin or fascia of the muscle is formed by connective tissue. Muscle is generally less echoic than subcutaneous fat or tendons. During contraction, the thickness of the body of the muscle increases, the echoic striae become more oblique, and the background becomes even more hypoechoic than at rest.

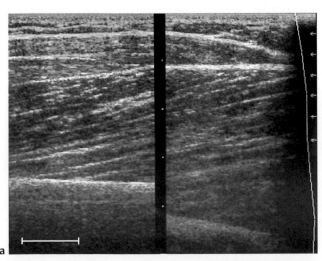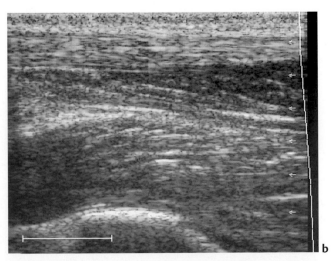

Fig. 20
Biceps muscle at rest and contracted (**a**). Musculotendinous junction (**b**).

Tendon

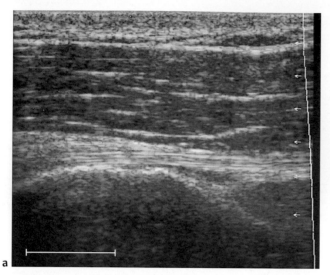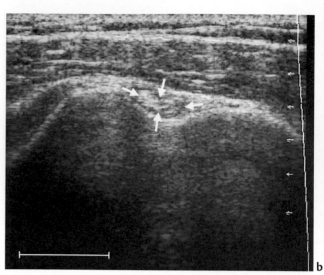

Fig. 21
Proximal biceps tendon shown in a longitudinal (**a**) and transverse scan (→) (**b**).

Normal tendons are homogeneous and highly echoic. Any slight obliquity of the beam may artifactually reduce this echogenicity and simulate tendinitis. A dynamic technique allows visualization of tendon movement. Images should be obtained in both the longitudinal and transverse planes. It is useful to scan the contralateral asymptomatic side of paired structures for comparison. The echogenicity of tendons is based upon their histological structure. Tendons are composed of longitudinally oriented bundles of collagen fibers. Some tendons, such as the biceps tendon, are surrounded by a synovial-lined sheath. These sheaths

are toroidal in shape, with a smooth synovial-lined inner surface, and contain a thin film of viscous mucoid fluid, which facilitates frictionless motion. The peritendon sheath creates a very thin, highly echoic line on either side of the tendon and is made of loose interstitial tissue. Other tendons, such as the Achilles tendon, do not possess a sheath and are surrounded by connective tissue forming the peritendon. These tendons are often accompanied by bursae at a site of friction. The insertion site can appear hypoechoic, due to its mixed fibrillar and cartilaginous nature and to anisotropy.

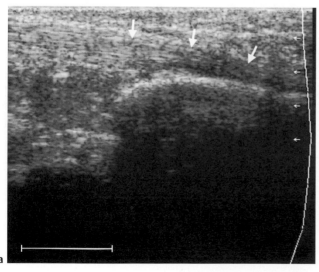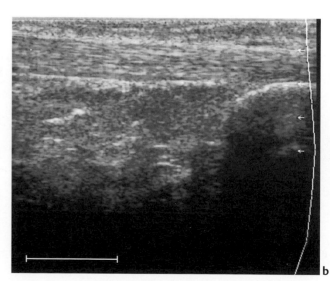

Fig. 22
Achilles tendon shown in a longitudinal view at the site of insertion (→) (**a**) and above (**b**).

Ligament

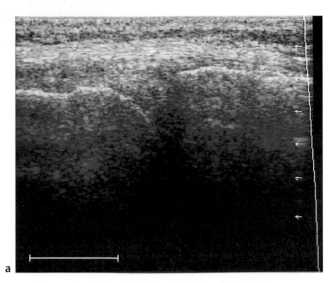
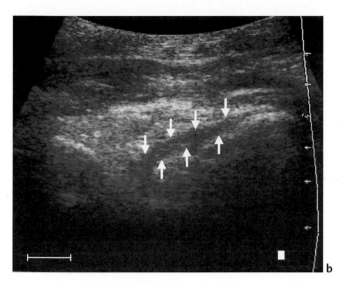

Fig. 23
Hyperechoic medial collateral ligament of the knee (→) (**a**). Hypoechoic posterior cruciate ligament of the knee (→) (**b**).

Extra-articular ligaments appear as hyperechoic bandlike structures. They are composed of dense collagen tissue and are extended from bone to bone. However, some ligaments, such as the lateral collateral ligament of the knee appear relatively hypoechoic. Intra-articular ligaments, such as the cruciate ligaments, show a hypoechoic structure. Ligaments are evaluated in a plane parallel to their long axis. On transverse scans, they are often indiscernible from the surrounding hyperechoic fat.

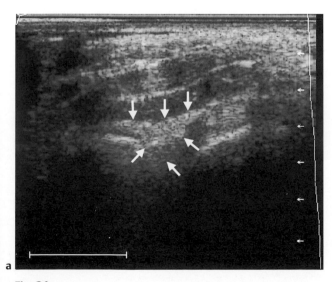
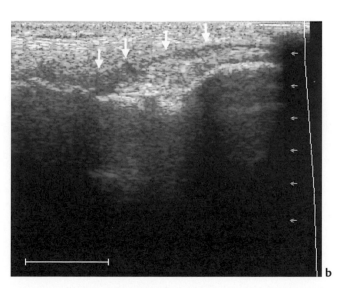

Fig. 24
Hyperechoic triangular carpal ligament (→) (**a**). Relatively hypoechoic lateral collateral ligament of the knee (→) (**b**).

Periosteum and Bone

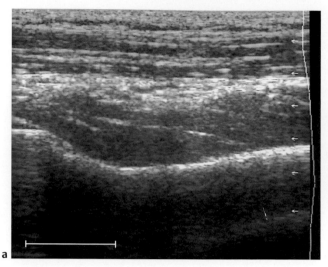 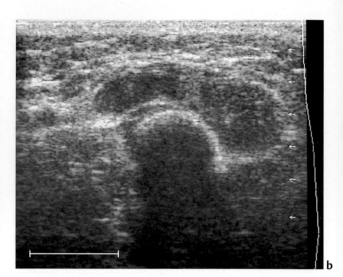

Fig. 25
Longitudinal (**a**) and transverse (**b**) scans of the proximal radius.

The proximal surface of the bone cortex appears on sonograms as a continuous smooth, densely reflective line. Bone interrupts the propagation of the ultrasound beam. The periosteum can only be visualized if abnormal. Detailed examination of the surface of cortical bone has applications in the evaluation of rheumatological diseases, trauma, and infection. Longitudinal and transverse examination should be perpendicular to the bone surface. Knowledge of the course of nutrient vessels allows them to be differentiated from fractures.

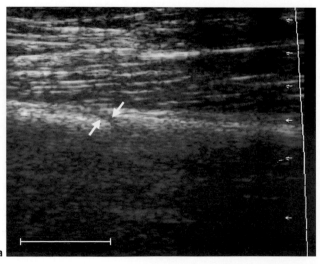 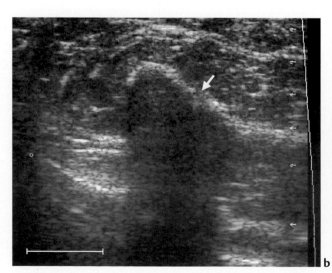

Fig. 26
Nutrient vessel (→) of the ulna in a longitudinal (**a**) and transverse (→) (**b**) scan.

Joint Capsule, Bursa, and Synovium

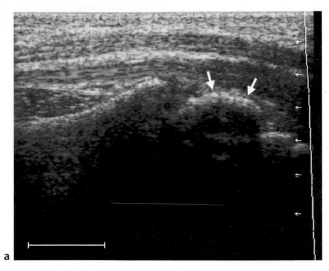
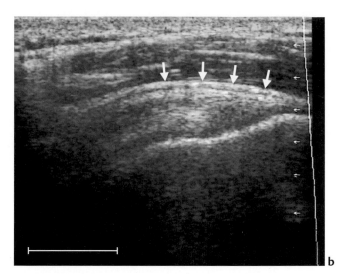

Fig. 27
Normal coxofemoral joint capsule (**a**). Normal subacromial-subdeltoid bursa (→) (**b**).

The joint capsule is visible as an echoic line. The periarticular ligaments, which contribute to the formation of the joint capsule are hyperechoic and inseparable from the inner surface of the capsule formed by a thin hypoechoic synovial layer. Bursae are synovial-lined sacs positioned between the tendon and the underlying bone. They facilitate frictionless motion, and are usually found adjacent to the tendon insertions. The subacromial-subdeltoid bursa is the largest in the body, covering the entire deep surface of the deltoid muscle. Some bursae communicate directly with the adjacent joint space, such as the suprapatellar bursa of the knee. However, most bursae are isolated and do not communicate with adjacent joints. Their walls are thin and hyperechoic, merging with the surrounding fat. The synovial inner layer is seen as a thin hypoechoic line.

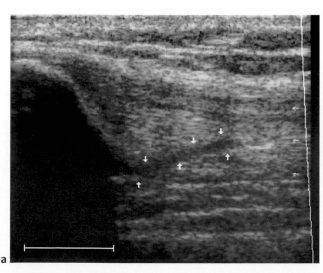
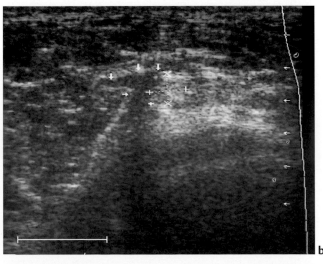

Fig. 28
Normal suprapatellar bursa (→) (**a**). Normal common gastrocnemius-semimembranosus bursa (→) (**b**).

Normal Appearances

Hyaline Cartilage

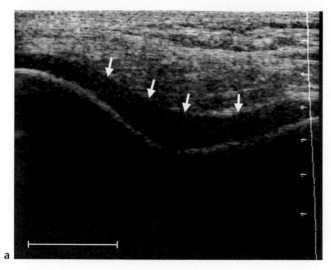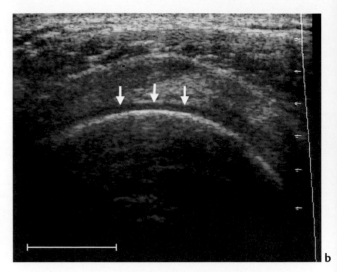

a   b

Fig. 29
Two examples of hyaline cartilage are shown with their typical hypoechoic appearance at the condylar groove (→) (**a**) and humeral head (→) (**b**).

The hypoechoic appearance of hyaline cartilage can be explained by the abundance of proteoglycans entrapping a large amount of water. Hyaline cartilage is present on the articular surface of synovial joints.

Fibrocartilage

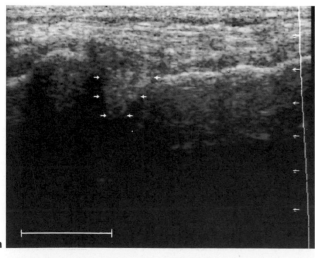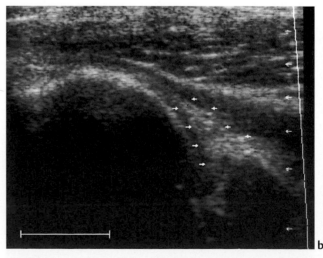

a   b

Fig. 30
The inner meniscus of the knee (→) (**a**) and the posterior labrum of the shoulder (→) (**b**) are composed of hyperechoic fibrocartilage.

The hyperechoic appearance of fibrocartilage can be explained by the greater amount and different orientation of collagen fibers in comparison to hyaline cartilage. Fibrocartilage is found in menisci and in tendinous and ligamentous attachments to bone.

Vessel

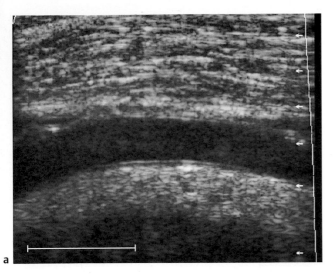 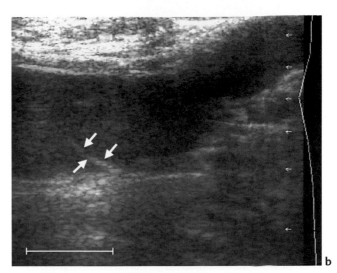

Fig. 31
Popliteal artery in a longitudinal plane (**a**). Hyperechoic valves of a femoral vein (→) (**b**).

Vessels have an anechoic round center on a transverse scan. The intimal layer can be distinguished as a fine hyperechoic line when using a high frequency probe. The media is hypoechoic and surrounded by a hyperechoic adventitia. Normal arteries are pulsatile. Superficial veins are thin walled and their caliber varies according to gravity or compression maneuvers. They may collapse under slight pressure of the probe. Venous anatomy shows many variants; typically, at least one vein accompanies the corresponding artery and has a larger diameter. Valves can be recognized as oblique hyperechoic structures in the venous lumen.

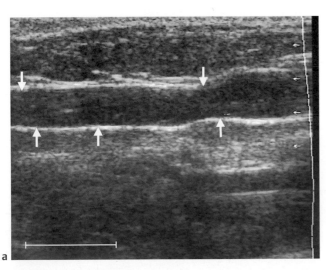 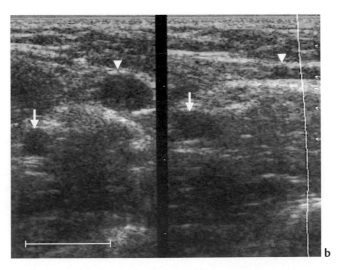

Fig. 32
Normal brachial artery (→) and basilar vein (▶) shown in a longitudinal (**a**) and a transverse scan (**b**). The lumen of the basilar vein disappears under compression.

Normal Appearances

Nerve

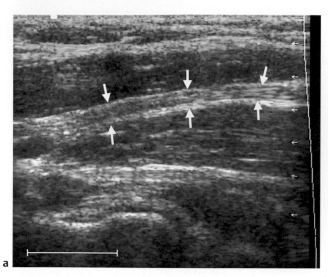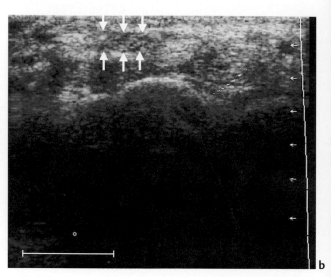

a   b

Fig. 33
Longitudinal scan of the ulnar nerve (→) at the level of the elbow (**a**). Transverse scan of the median nerve (→) (**b**).

The normal nerves appear as hyperechoic tubular structures. On longitudinal scans, the echostructure is fibrillar, similar to that of tendons. On transverse scans, the hyperechoic nerves contain small cystlike formations and may simulate ovarian morphology. Fascicles of nerve fibers appear as hypoechoic cystlike formations and are surrounded by a hyperechoic perineurium. The outer envelope of the nerve is composed of hyperechoic collagenous tissue, called the epineurium. In contrast to tendons, nerves cannot be mobilized and show less anisotropy. In the upper extremity, sonography can routinely identify the median nerve in the forearm and carpal tunnel, the radial nerve in the arm and at the elbow, and the ulnar nerve at the elbow and in the forearm. In the lower extremity, the sciatic nerve is visible in the posterior thigh; the tibial and popliteal nerves can be seen in the popliteal fossa.

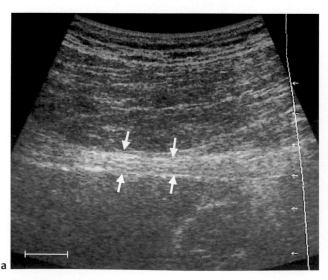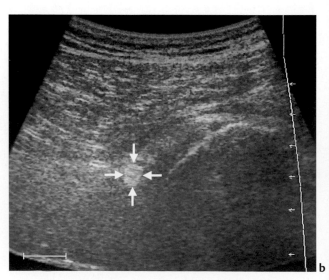

a   b

Fig. 34
Longitudinal (**a**) and transverse (**b**) scan of the sciatic nerve (→) in the posterior thigh.

Fat and Skin

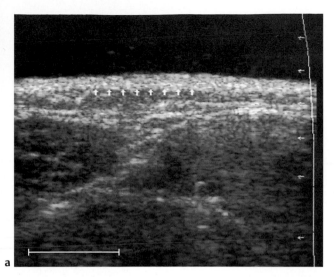
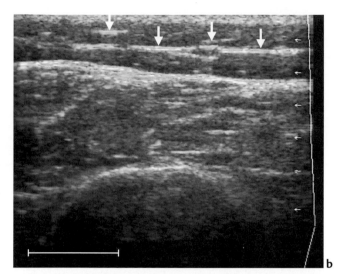

Fig. 35
Hyperechoic normal skin (→) (**a**). Normal hypoechoic subcutaneous fat with hyperechoic fibrous bands (→) (**b**).

The subcutaneous tissue is composed mainly of fat, which is hypoechoic and contains linear echoes corresponding to strands of connective tissue. The echogenicity and the thickness change from patient to patient and with topography. The skin should be evaluated with a high frequency transducer. It appears as a regular layer with variable thickness, which ranges from 1.4 to 4.8 mm depending on the examined region. The epidermis and dermis cannot be differentiated. Skin appendages can be studied with high frequency adapted transducers (15–20 MHz). The skin is thicker in men than in women.

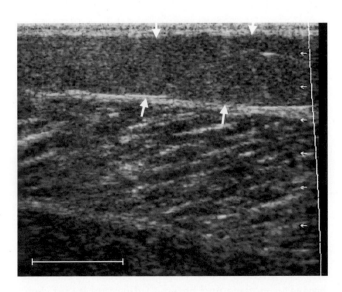

Fig. 36
Normal hyperechoic subcutaneous fat (→).

Basic Signs of Pathology: Muscle

Hypertrophy

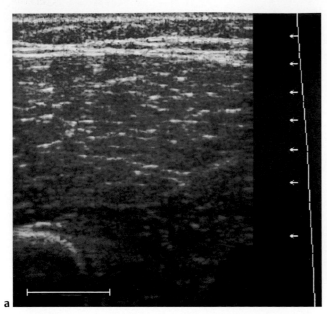
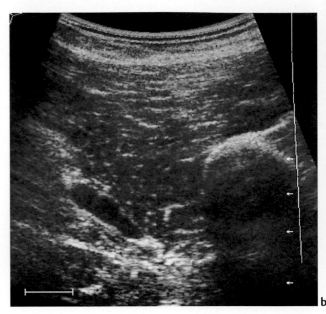

Fig. 37
Transverse scan of a hypertrophied quadriceps muscle evaluated with a 7.5 MHz (**a**) and a 5 MHz (**b**) transducer.

Since muscle bundles are hypoechoic and separated by hyperechoic fibro-adipose septae, a hypertrophied muscle will demonstrate global decreased echogenicity. The same phenomenon appears during contrac- tion. Hypertrophy is frequently encountered in athletes; its appearance may be simulated after excercise lasting several minutes.

Atrophy

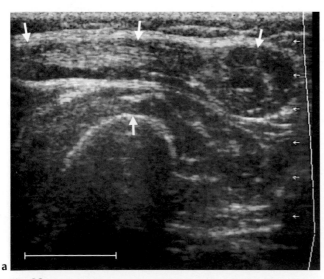
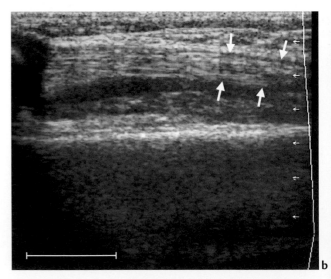

Fig. 38
Transverse and longitudinal scan of the quadriceps muscle show advanced atrophy (→). Notice the muscular thinning and hyperechoic echo texture (**a** and **b**).

In generalized muscle atrophy, the muscle bundles decrease in volume and become infiltrated by fat, leading to increased echogenicity. Muscle atrophy can be focal. When secondary to trauma, fibrosis can result in retraction of septae and fascias. Atrophy is best seen on CT or MRI.

Elongation

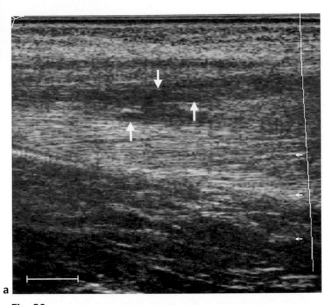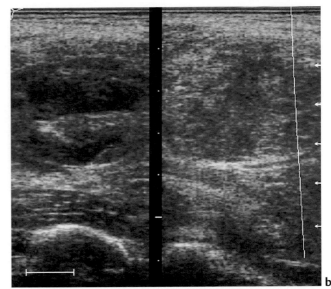

Fig. 39
An elongation injury to the rectus femoris muscle shows a discrete rupture of the pennate structure on a longitudinal scan (→) (**a**) and a heterogeneous, speckled, microcystic appearance on a transverse scan (**b**).

Elongation is the first stage of a muscle distraction injury. It consists of microruptures that produce an echographic microcystic pattern on a transverse scan. On a longitudinal scan, the microruptures have an elongated appearance and resemble small lakes. Elongation injury involves less than five percent of the muscular cross-sectional area, as seen on a transverse section.

Partial Rupture

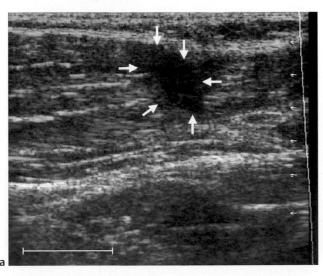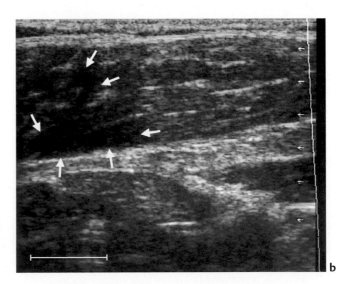

Fig. 40
Two partial muscle ruptures show an anechoic collection (→), filling in the gap between the ruptured fiber bundles (**a** and **b**).

Partial rupture is also due to a distraction mechanism. It appears as a gap or a hypoechoic collection in the muscle, with loss of continuity of the fibers. This differentiates partial rupture from simple elongation. The contraction of the muscle allows differentiation between an echoic clot and the ruptured muscle.

Basic Signs of Pathology: Muscle

Complete Rupture

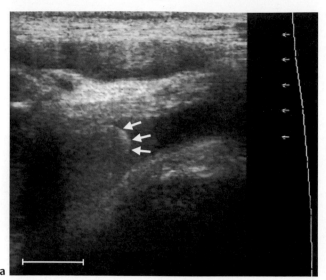
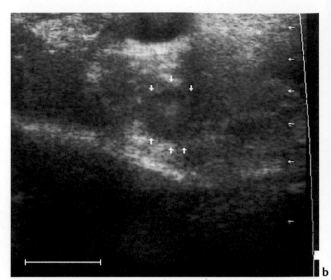

Fig. 41
A complete rupture of the distal part of the iliopsoas muscle is seen in a longitudinal plane, showing the rounded muscle end (bell-clapper sign) (→) lying between the femoral vessels and the anterior acetabular rim (**a**). The transverse plane shows the muscular stump surrounded by the hematoma (halo sign) (→) (**b**).

In complete rupture, there is a clear cut separation of the muscle belly by the hematoma. The bell-clapper sign is present: a rounded aspect of the retracted muscle surrounded by the hematoma. There is total functional loss. Complete rupture is less frequent than partial rupture. On transverse sections, there is a halo or target sign that corresponds to the cross-section of the retracted muscle surrounded by the hematoma.

Hematoma

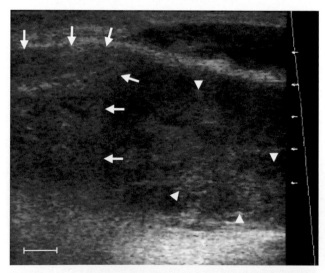
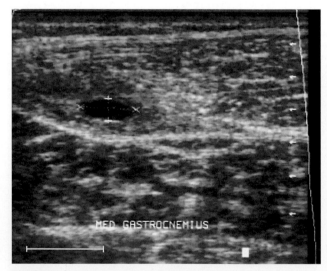

Fig. 42
Hyperechoic hematoma (▶) in the quadriceps muscle.

Fig. 43
Small anechoic rupture in the calf muscle two days after blunt injury (→).

In the acute phase, hematomas are hyperechoic and show an echogenicity similar to that of muscle. Small partial ruptures are more accurately detected 24 to 48 hours after injury. The hyperechogenicity disappears within three days, and dissolved clots become anecho-ic. The subsequent organization of the hematoma results in generation of internal echoes, dispersed throughout the collection. Because of continued clot lysis, late hematomas contain fewer internal echoes, and return to an anechoic pattern.

Crush Injury

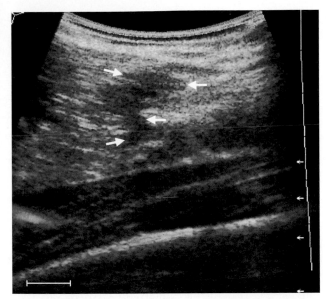

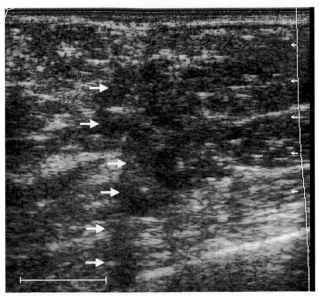

Fig. 44
Rupture of the vastus lateralis muscle, with irregular borders and a ruptured aponeurosis (→), in a soccer player who had experienced a direct impact.

Fig. 45
Crush injury in a 50-year-old woman who had had a car accident. Irregular muscular disruption is seen in the vastus lateralis muscle and in the vastus intermedius muscle on this coronal image (→).

Muscle crush injury is caused by blunt trauma. The muscle fibers are compressed against the bone, resulting in the destruction of a large number of fibers and in hematoma formation. In crush injury, the fascias can also be ruptured, as the injury may affect several adjacent muscles. Crush injury appears as a cavity with irregular borders. Its contents are echoic. The hematoma is difficult to evaluate, but becomes anechoic after a few days. About 20% of these injuries induce myositis ossificans.

Delayed-Onset Muscle Soreness

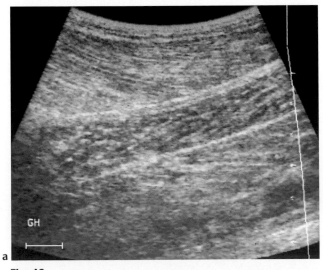

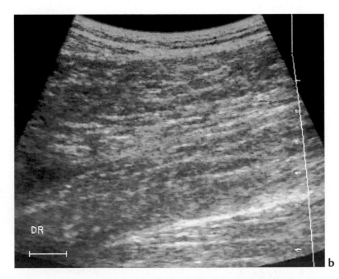

a

b

Fig. 46
This patient presented with a persistent pain in the calf, after a six-hour intensive tennis session the day before. The muscles appeared swollen and hyperechoic (**a**) in comparison to the normal side (**b**). No fiber interruption was noted.

Edema can be due to trauma, but also to ischemia, infarction, or infection. It results in increased echogenicity, obscuring the normal pennate structure of the muscle. Delayed-onset muscle soreness corresponds to muscle edema following exercise. It persists after the strain, causing pain or cramps.

Healing

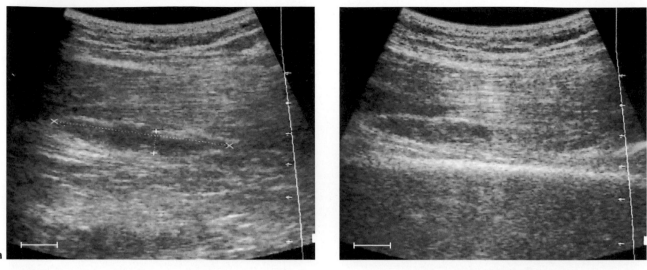

a   b

Fig. 47
Longitudinal scan of the vastus externus muscle, showing a partial rupture during healing. There is an interval of three weeks between the two scans.

Ultrasound is useful for following the evolution of muscular rupture. Healing of muscle tears occurs usually between the third and the sixteenth week. Duration depends on the extent and location of the lesion. During the healing process, muscle ruptures gradually fill in with granulation tissue, seen as fine nodular echoic structures at the periphery of the lesion. This echoic band thickens progressively, and eventually totally replaces the cavity. Finally, a lamellar scar can be seen as a hyperechoic band, sometimes accompanied by acoustic shadows.

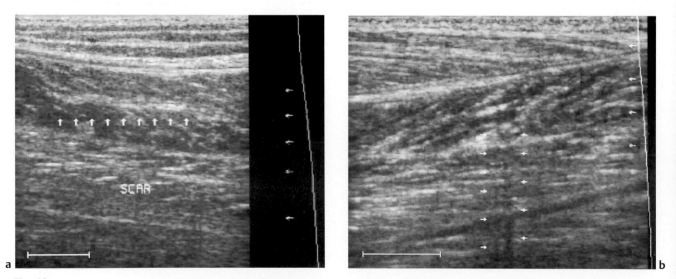

a   b

Fig. 48
A scar seen as a linear hyperechoic band (→) in the gastrocnemius muscle in a longitudinal (**a**) and a transverse plane (**b**). The latter scar shows a posterior shadow (→), despite the absence of calcifications.

Healing Complications

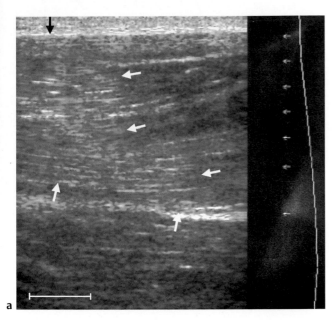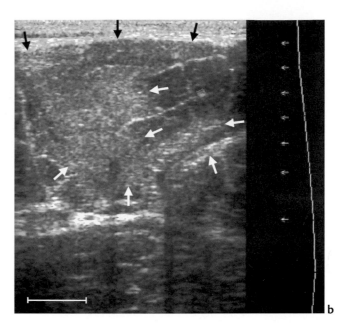

Fig. 49
Muscular fibrosis is defined by a diffuse hyperechoic echotexture surrounded by normal muscle. Muscular fibrosis (→) was found in the biceps femoris of this karate instructor in a longitudinal (**a**) and transverse (**b**) scan.

Complications of healing are fibrosis, calcifications, myositis ossificans, and cyst formation. In fibrosis, the muscle fibers appear hyperechoic. Another sign of fibrosis is retraction of fascias and septae, indicating loss of muscular volume. Muscular fibers remain continuous. Calcifications appear as hyperechoic foci, sometimes accompanied by an acoustic shadow. A cyst is a rare complication of muscle healing, and can cause local pain.

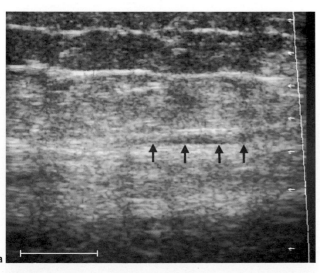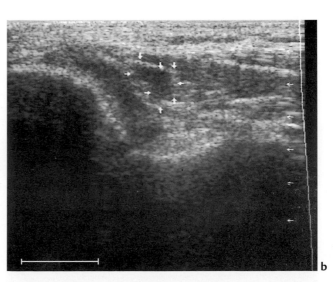

Fig. 50
Muscular fibrosis predisposes to rupture (→) (**a**) due to diminished elasticity. This patient was immobilized for only 10 days after a partial rupture of the pronator teres muscle. The transverse scan (**b**) was made 2.5 years after this event, and shows a cyst-like formation (→), explaining persistent pain.

Basic Signs of Pathology: Muscle

Myositis Ossificans

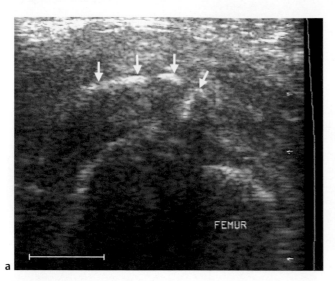

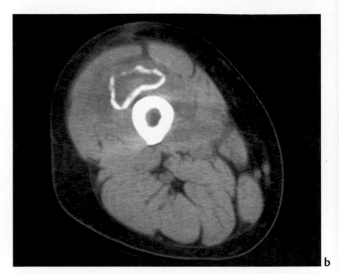

Fig. 51
Myositis ossificans of the vastus intermedius muscle presenting as a mass with peripheral calcifications and hypoechoic content (→) (**a**). Corresponding CT (**b**).

Myositis ossificans may be post-traumatic (60–75%), idiopathic, or develop as a consequence of general diseases such as burns or neurological conditions. Preferential locations are the elbow, thigh, and buttocks. Histologically, the core of the lesion is composed of proliferating fibroblasts and areas of hemorrhage and necrosis. In the intermediate zone, osteoblasts and islands of immature bone are seen. The peripheral zone is characterized by the presence of native bone trabeculae. The appearance of the lesion changes over time. The initial pattern is an ill-defined soft-tissue mass without calcifications, usually hypoechoic. Over time, ossifications and calcifications appear at the periphery of the lesion. Maturation of the lesion takes five to six months. There are two important differences from periosteal sarcomas: there is no mass beyond the calcification, and the periosteum is usually normal.

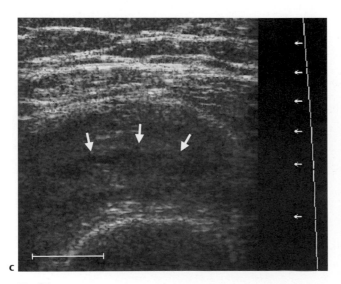

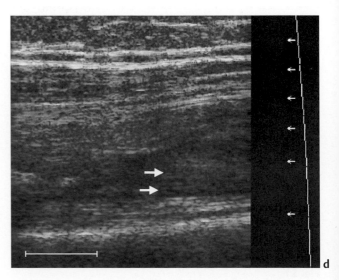

Fig. 51
At the periphery, muscle fibers can be seen penetrating this myositis ossificans shown in a transverse (→) (**c**) and longitudinal (→) (**d**) scan, allowing a correct diagnosis even in the absence of peripheral calcifications.

Compartment Syndrome

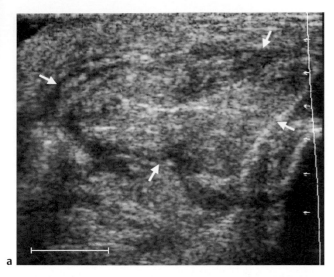
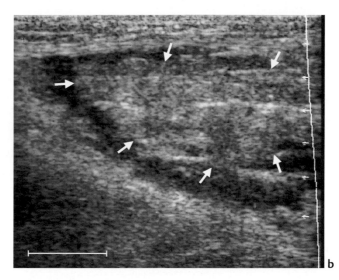

Fig. 52
Posterior transverse scans of the left calf show a hyperechoic muscular structure (→) with normal-looking fibers located close to the fascia (**a** and **b**).

In acute compartment syndrome, ultrasound shows a diffuse increase in echogenicity, while the peripheral muscle bundles remain hypoechoic. The volume of the compartment is also increased, and the fascias bulge, as does the interosseous membrane. At a later stage, rhabdomyolysis occurs and a heterogeneous ultrasound appearance results, with anechoic or hypoechoic collections. Muscle necrosis leads to fibrosis and ossification. At the stage of necrosis, the evolution is irreversible.

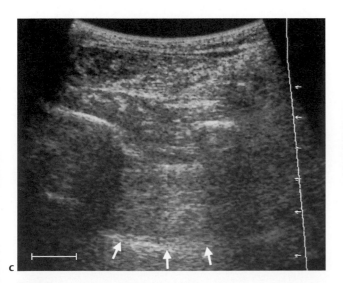
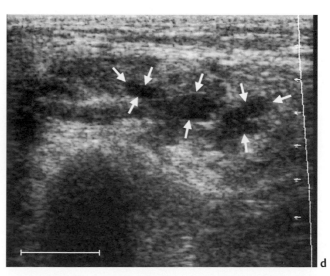

Fig. 52
Swelling of the superficial and deep muscles of the calf causes anterior bulging of the interosseous membrane (→) (**c**). Heterogeneous muscle in a compartment syndrome with formation of cystic zones (→) corresponds to necrosis due to rhabdomyolysis (**d**).

Basic Signs of Pathology: Muscle

Accessory Muscle

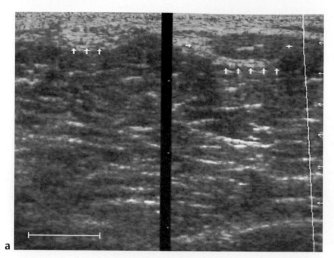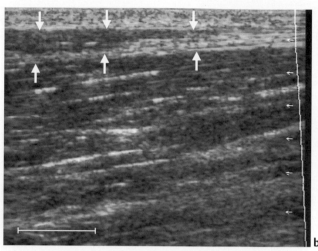

Fig. 53
Ultrasound reveals an accessory muscle belly running parallel to the posterior surface of the semimembranous muscle in the upper thigh (→) (**a**). A longitudinal scan demonstrates the superficial position of the musculotendinous junction (→) (**b**). The patient complained of tension in the posterior aspect of the thigh and knee.

Accessory muscles are rare. The best known is the accessory soleus muscle, which inserts into the upper or medial surface of the calcaneum. Accessory muscles are often symptomatic, and appear as painful masses, particularly when overused, as in ballet dancers.

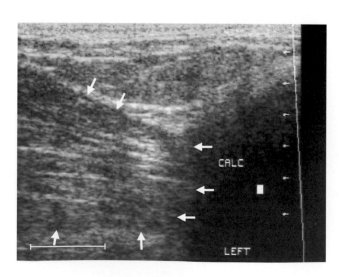

Fig. 54
An accessory soleus muscle (→) inserting on the upper aspect of the calcaneum in this dancer, who complained of a painful mass at the ankle when she exercised.

Herniation

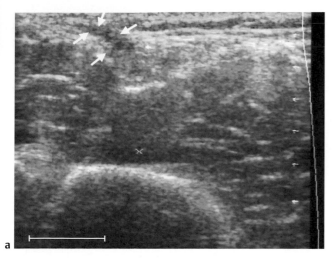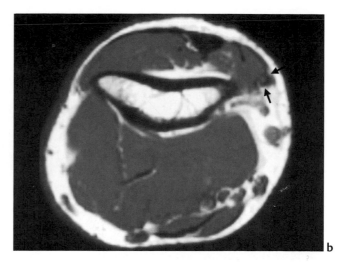

Fig. 55
This athlete felt a small nodule, which swelled and became painful during exercise, at the anteromedial border of the triceps, proximal to the elbow. Ultrasound showed a ruptured fascia and a small muscle herniation (→) (**a**). The corresponding T_1-weighted magnetic resonance image showed the same finding in this axial plane (→) (**b**).

Muscle herniation appears as a local swelling protruding through a ruptured fascia. The small herniated nodule has the same echogenicity as the adjacent muscle. It is better seen with muscle contraction, which accentuates the bulging of the herniation.

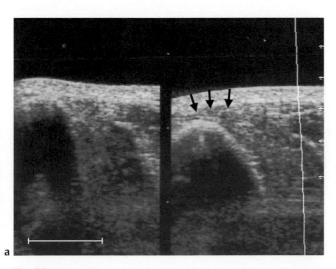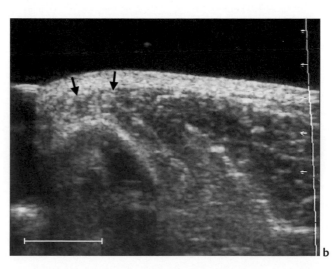

Fig. 56
The anterior tibial muscle herniates in front of the anterior tibial aspect, as seen in a comparative study (→) (**a**) and accentuated by contraction (→) (**b**).

Basic Signs of Pathology: Tendon

Acute Tendinitis

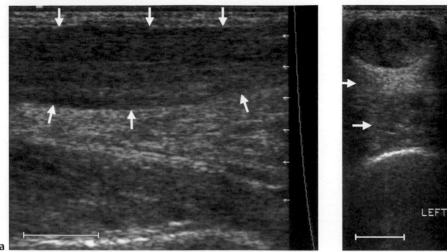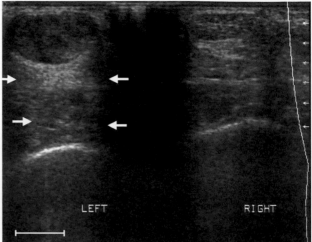

Fig. 57
Longitudinal (**a**) and comparative transverse (**b**) scan of a thickened, hypoechoic Achilles tendon (→) with posterior acoustic enhancement.

In tendons without a synovial sheath, acute tendinitis appears as thickening of the tendon, with global or focal hypoechogenicity. Focal hypoechoic areas may simulate a partial rupture, but have a limited longitudinal extent. Posterior enhancement and lateral shadows due to refraction are present especially on axial scans. In tendons with synovial sheaths, the tendon can thicken, but remains hyperechoic. Tendinitis is accompanied by tenosynovitis, with an increased amount of fluid in the synovial sheath. On transverse sonograms, the fluid gives a target image, with an anechoic halo around the tendon. On longitudinal sonograms, anechoic lines surround the tendon. The fluid is easier to see on transverse scans, because excessive compression shifts it away on longitudinal views. The fluid can become echoic in traumatic tenosynovitis.

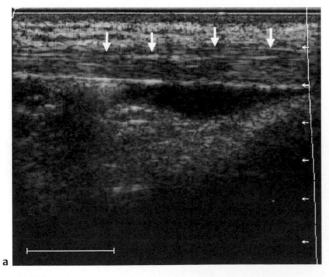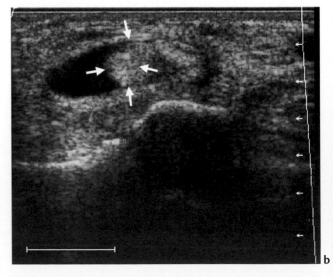

Fig. 58
Longitudinal (**a**) and transverse scans (**b**) show a thickened posterior tibial tendon (→) and a distended, fluidfilled tendon sheath in this patient with tendinitis and tenosynovitis.

Chronic Tendinitis

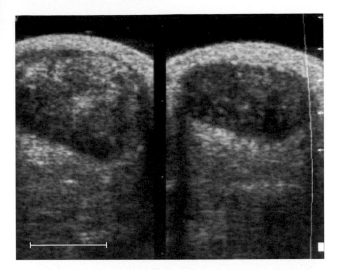

Fig. 59
Axial scans of an Achilles tendon that appears thickened, hypoechoic, and nodular.

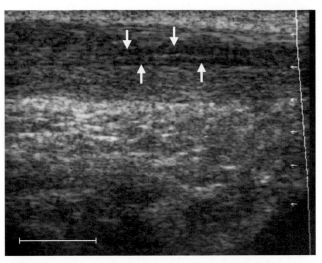

Fig. 60
Linear fissures (→) are seen in this tendinitis of the Achilles tendon.

In tendons without a synovial sheath, chronic tendinitis shows global or, more often, focal thickening, with heterogeneous echogenicity. The tendon may have a nodular appearance and irregular and ill-defined borders. Ultrasound also shows microruptures of the tendons. These pathologic findings can be present in the acute and chronic forms of tendinitis, which should be considered as a continuous spectrum of the same disease. The tendon insertion can be calcified, and sometimes calcium deposits are present within the tendon. They are present as hyperechoic foci, sometimes accompanied by an acoustic shadow, and are pathognomonic for chronic tendinitis. In tendons with a synovial sheath, irregular hypoechoic or hyperechoic thickening of the synovium is present, with or without fluid.

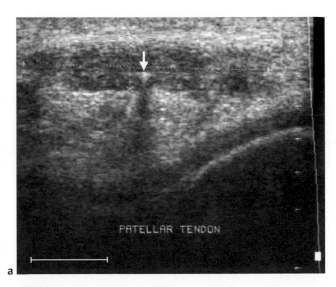

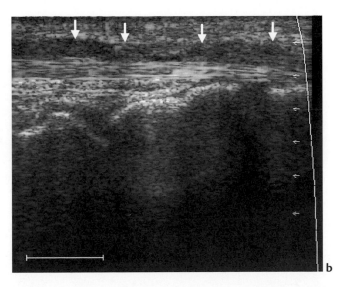

Fig. 61
Calcifications (→) in a nodular chronic patellar tendinitis, pathognomonic of chronicity (**a**). Diffuse irregular synovial thickening (→) in a chronic tenosynovitis of an anterior tibial tendon (**b**).

Tendinitis, Miscellaneous

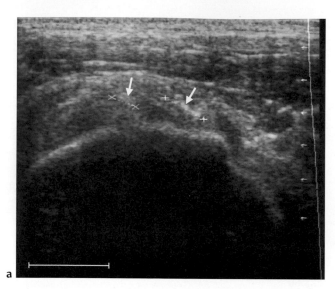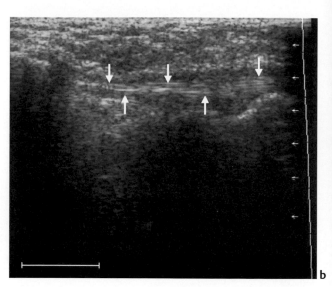

Fig. 62
Calcified tendinitis of the rotator cuff is shown in this axial scan, giving the cuff a heterogeneous appearance (→) (**a**). A hypoechoic pannus partially destroys the extensor carpi ulnaris tendon (→) (**b**).

Metabolic and systemic disorders can induce various types of tendinitis. Calcifying tendinitis occurs frequently in the shoulder and wrist, due to hydroxyapatite deposits. Calcifications can cause false images of tears. In hemodialysis patients, amyloid deposits cause thickening and heterogenicity of the tendon. In rheumatoid arthritis, hypoechoic pannus tends to destroy the tendons. Goutty tophi are less destructive, and have a heterogeneous nodular echo texture.

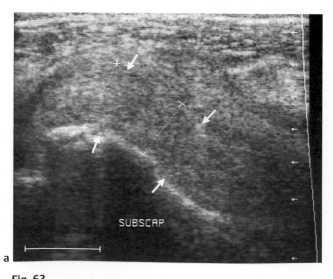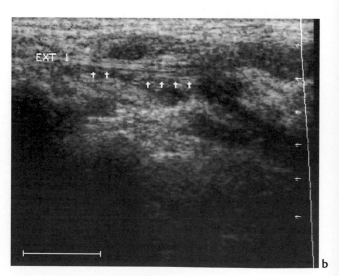

Fig. 63
This chronic hemodialysis patient presented with a thickened heterogeneous subscapularis tendon due to amyloid deposit (→) (**a**). A tophus of mixed echogenicity surrounds the extensor pollicis longus tendon (→) (**b**).

Partial Rupture

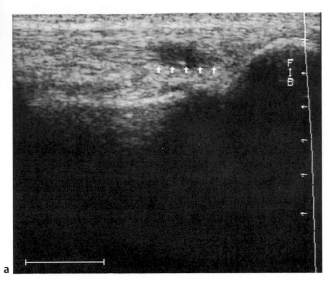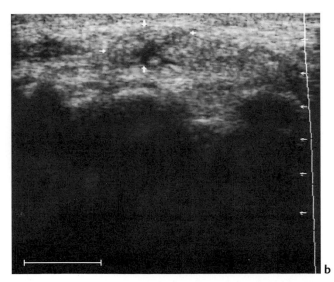

Fig. 64
Longitudinal (**a**) and axial (**b**) scans of a partial biceps tendon rupture (→) close to its insertion on the fibular head, giving an anechoic gap in the tendon substance.

The appearance of tendon rupture is variable, depending on the site and the presence or absence of a synovial sheath. In partial rupture, anechoic clefts are seen within the tendon, with interruption of fibers and increased synovial fluid within the sheath. A partial rupture of a tendon without a synovial sheath results in localized thickening of the tendon, a defect of the tendon contour with interruption of fibers, and fluid filling the clefts within the tendon. The end result is either a defect or a hypoechoic, localized thickening of the tendon, which extends over a considerable distance in a longitudinal plane.

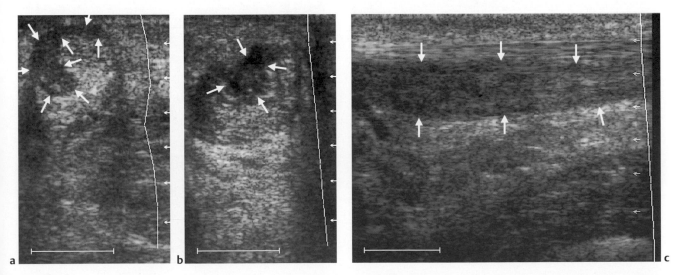

Fig. 65
A partial rupture of the Achilles tendon in a transverse scan is seen as a crescent-shaped, hypoechoic thickening (→) (**a**) or as a fluid-filled defect (→) (**b**). The hypoechoic anterior part of the Achilles tendon (→) in a longitudinal scan indicates partial rupture (**c**).

Basic Signs of Pathology: Tendon

Complete Rupture

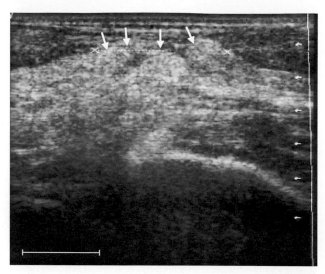

Fig. 66
Complete rupture of the Achilles tendon at the musculotendinous junction. Fat is herniating into the tendon gap (→).

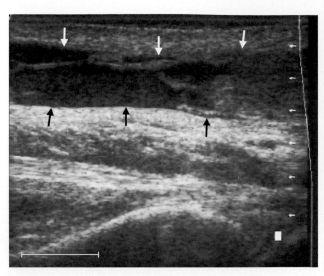

Fig. 67
An anechoic hematoma replaces the Achilles tendon in a complete rupture (→).

A complete rupture of a tendon with a synovial sheath results in an empty sheath, with fluid separating the retracted ends. Ultrasound also shows longitudinal ruptures as anechoic clefts, separating the ends of the tendon, which are usually thickened and surrounded by a distended sheath. In a tendon without a synovial sheath, an interruption of all fibers with retraction of the ends is seen, with a hematoma or fat filling the gap, particularly in the Achilles tendon. The rounded aspect of the retracted ends can induce a refraction artifact.

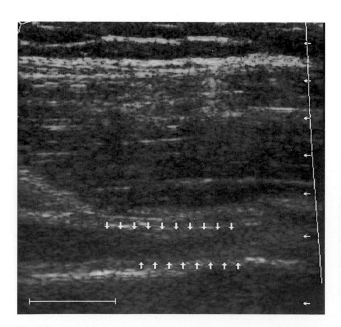

Fig. 68
The biceps tendon is absent in its fluid-filled sheath (→).

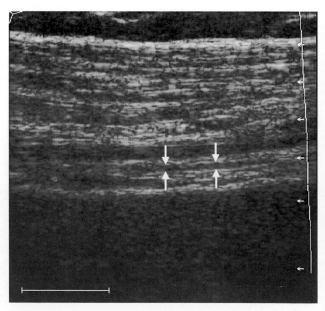

Fig. 69
A longitudinal hypoechoic rupture of the bicipital tendon, with a distended sheath (→).

Injury

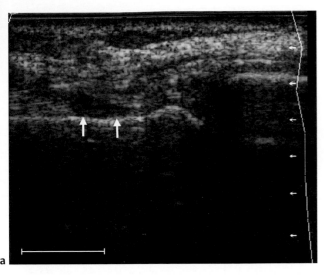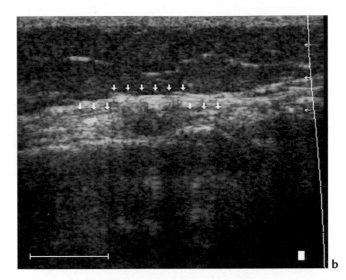

Fig. 70
A complete rupture of the medial collateral ligament is present, with interruption of the superficial and deep parts visible as a hypoechoic gap (→) (**a**). A partial rupture of the medial collateral ligament (deep layer) is seen (→) (**b**). The overlying hyperechoic superficial part is intact.

Sonography is of particular interest in the examination of the extra-articular ligaments, and is best performed in a longitudinal plane, parallel to the long axis of the ligament. In sprain, the ligament is thickened and hypoechoic. In partial or complete rupture, the hyperechoic band is partially or completely ruptured, with a hematoma filling the cleft, which can appear hypoechoic or anechoic. Retraction of the ends of the ligament can be seen. Healing occurs slowly. After several months, the ligament regains its normal appearance. In fact, a favorable evolution can be observed if adequate treatment has been applied. Unfavorable evolution can take two forms: a persistent interruption of the ligament, or a hypertrophic repair, appearing as a tender hypoechoic mass of granulation tissue within the hyperechoic ligament. Sometimes calcifications are present. Normal intra-articular ligaments are hypoechoic. They thicken or become discontinuous when torn.

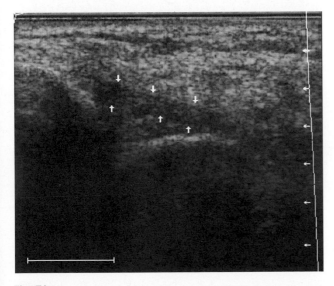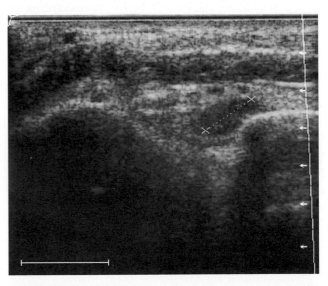

Fig. 71
A hypoechoic anterior tibiofibular ligament in this case of ankle sprain (→).

Fig. 72
A rounded hypoechoic tender nodule in an untreated partial rupture of an anterior tibiofibular ligament.

Basic Signs of Pathology: Bursa

Acute Bursitis

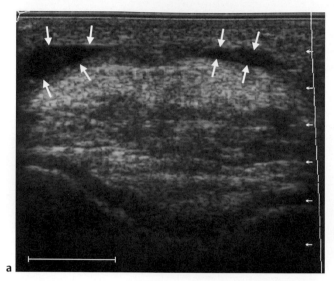
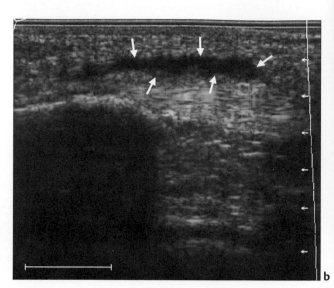

Fig. 73
A painful superior prepatellar bursitis (→) is shown in an axial (**a**) and sagittal (**b**) plane as a fluid-filled and easily depressed sac-like structure.

In case of acute bursitis, ultrasound shows an increased volume of the bursa, with an anechoic content. The wall of the bursa remains thin, which differentiates the acute from the chronic form. Typical localizations are prepatellar, deep infrapatellar, or retrocalcaneal bursitis. Acute bursitis can be of inflammatory, infectious, or frictional origin.

Chronic Bursitis

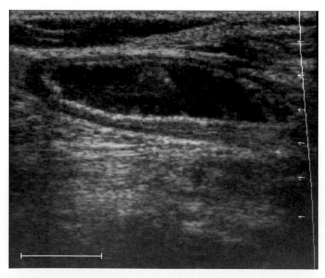
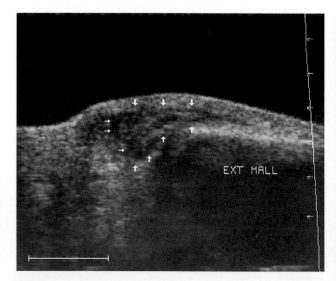

Fig. 74
A thickened wall is a sign of chronicity as shown in this Baker's cyst.

Fig. 75
A de novo bursitis of frictional origin has a chronic thick wall (→) as shown in this inframalleolar location.

Chronic bursitis results from repetitive friction over a long period of time. The wall of the bursa becomes thickened, and the content can be anechoic, hypo-echoic, or hyperechoic. The outline of the bursa is irregular and indistinct. Newly formed or de novo bursitis is always of the chronic type.

Inflammatory and Infectious Bursitis

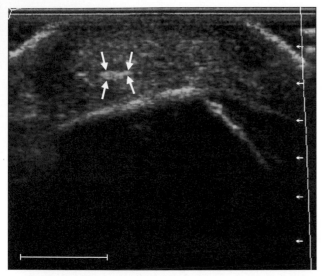

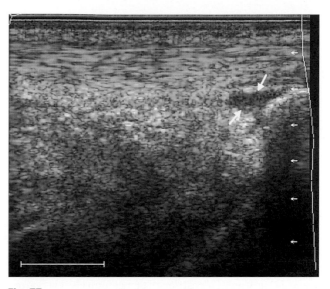

Fig. 76
The homogeneous echoic content seen in this olecranon bursitis corresponds to pus surrounding a fragmented hyperechoic wooden foreign body (→).

Fig. 77
A retrocalcaneal bursitis (→) in a young man with ankylosing spondylitis.

Inflammatory bursitis can occur in systemic diseases such as rheumatoid arthritis or ankylosing spondylitis. The wall of the bursa is thickened and the content has a variable appearance, often containing sparse echoes. Septic bursitis most commonly appears in the olecranon and prepatellar bursa. The content is homogeneously echoic, and the wall is thickened.

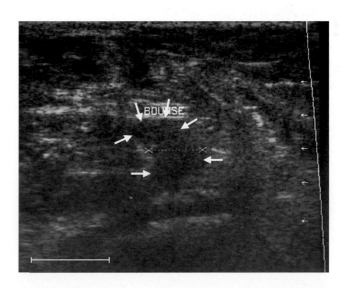

Fig. 78
Synovial thickening (→) in a common gastrocnemius-semimembranosus bursa, tender on palpation, in a patient with rheumatoid arthritis. There was no associated Baker's cyst.

Basic Signs of Pathology: Bursa

Hemorrhagic Bursitis

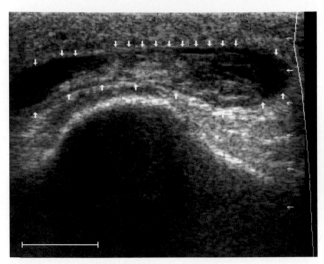

Fig. 79
A transverse scan of a posttraumatic hemorrhagic inferior patellar bursitis (→) in front of the tibial tuberosity, with clots of mixed echogenicity and contusional edema in the surrounding subcutaneous fat.

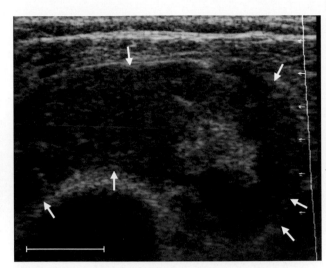

Fig. 80
Hemorrhagic subdeltoideal bursitis (→) in a dialysis patient.

Hemorrhagic bursitis can have many causes, such as direct trauma, rupture of an adjacent tendon, or bone fracture and bleeding disorders. The bursa appears more distended than in frictional bursitis. The fluid contains echoes, but the global appearance varies over time. Immediately after trauma, the bursa contains echoic material that settles in the lower part. Later on, the contents become heterogeneous, with irregular hyperechoic masses, corresponding to blood clots, floating in fluid. There is no thickening of the synovial wall.

Metabolic Bursitis

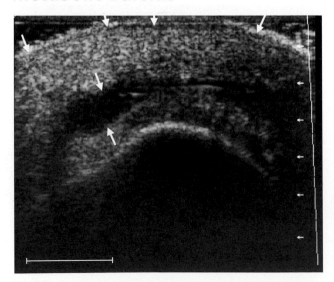

Fig. 81
In an acute inferior patellar bursitis in a patient with gout, anechoic contents are associated with severe peribursal inflammation (→).

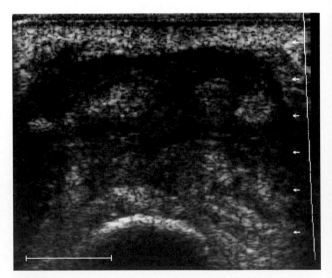

Fig. 82
In the chronic form, the fluid becomes echoic, and hyperechoic nodules and septations are present.

The most common cause of metabolic bursitis is gout. In the first stage, the contents may be anechoic, but in chronic forms, the contents become echoic and heterogeneous, with hyperechoic nodules, sometimes calcifications and septae. Edema spreads into the surrounding fat, which appears more echoic.

Effusion

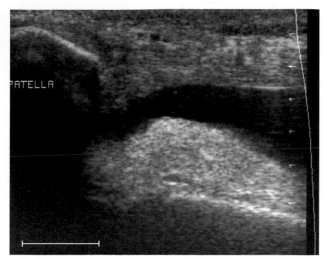

Fig. 83
Anechoic effusion in a longitudinal scan of the suprapatellar pouch in this patient with chondromalacia.

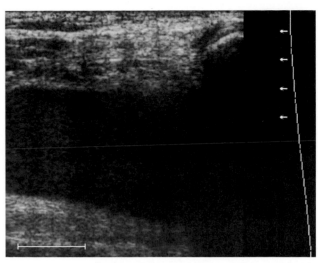

Fig. 84
A homogeneous hypoechoic effusion in the suprapatellar pouch corresponds to hemarthrosis.

Ultrasound is an appropriate method for detecting effusions, since small volumes of fluid can be seen. Intra-articular fluid is a nonspecific finding, and accompanies a great variety of joint diseases: degenerative, traumatic, inflammatory, or tumoral. A specific diagnosis can only be made on the basis of an aspiration. The echogenicity of the fluid varies with its composition and the cause of the effusion. In simple effusion, as in transient synovitis of the hip in children, the fluid is anechoic or hypoechoic. In septic arthritis, a diffusely echoic fluid, thickening of the joint capsule, and irregularities of the synovium are seen. In hemarthrosis and lipohemarthrosis, the fluid is hypoechoic, with some echoic masses corresponding to blood clots or fat lobules.

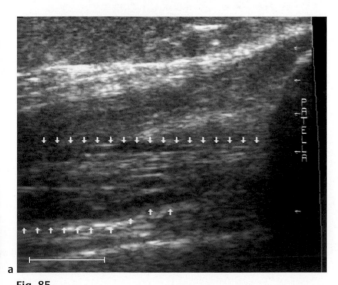

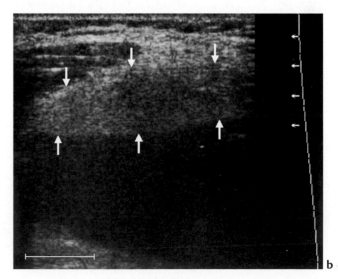

Fig. 85
Longitudinal (**a**) and transvserse (**b**) scans of lipohemarthrosis in patients with tibial plateau fracture. Hyperechoic fat is floating on the surface of the effusion (→). The echoic fluid under the fat lobules reflects hemarthrosis. Blood, when clotted, can also form depressible nodules.

Basic Signs of Pathology: Capsule

Septic Effusion

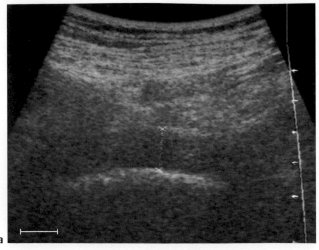

Fig. 86
Transverse (**a**) and sagittal (**b**) scan of a septic effusion in the hip.

In septic arthritis, the effusion appears homogeneously hypoechoic. Occasionally, the contents can have an echogenicity similar to that of muscle. Fluid aspiration can be guided with ultrasound control.

Loose bodies

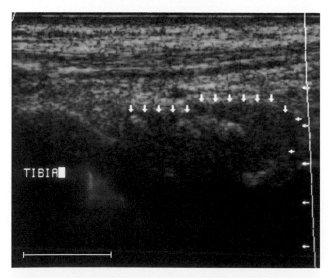

Fig. 87
A distended anterior recess (→) of the subtalar joint containing multiple fragments shown in the sagittal plane.

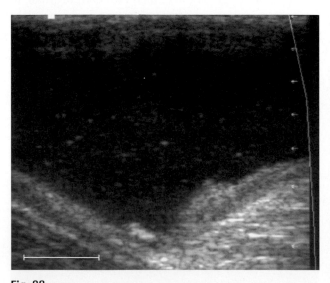

Fig. 88
Hyperechoic foci in this Baker's cyst with a thickened wall correspond to cholesterol cristals after corticoid injection.

Ultrasound is an excellent method of detecting loose bodies (see also the sections on elbow, knee, and ankle). Loose bodies have a variable origin and composition made of fibrin, villi, cartilage, and cristals. They appear as hyperechoic foci, floating in the effusion, or embedded in the synovial wall. They are often concentrated in synovial recesses. Cartilage fragments can calcify. An acoustic shadow is an occasional finding.

Synovial Thickening

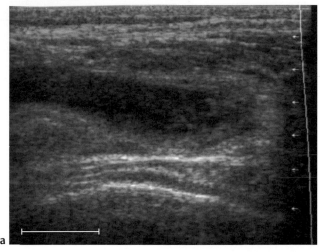 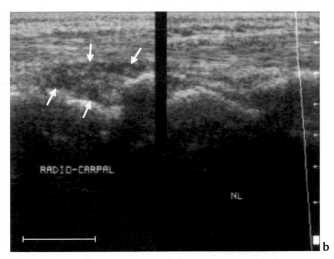

Fig. 89
Synovial thickening is seen as a hypoechoic wall in the suprapatellar recess in a patient with rheumatoid arthritis. Notice the presence of echoes within the fluid, due to its highly cellular composition or debris (**a**). Synovial thickening (→) in the radiocarpal joint is seen in this comparative longitudinal scan (**b**).

The synovial wall can become thickened in many situations. A diffuse, regular thickening is seen in inflammatory or infectious diseases. In rheumatoid arthritis, thickening is diffuse, but may show nodules. In pigmented villonodular synovitis (PVNS), focal thickening is present. The synovium can contain calcifications, as in osteochondromatosis, or after steroid injection. The synovial wall usually appears hypoechoic, and measurements of its thickness are obtained by compression of the articular recess.

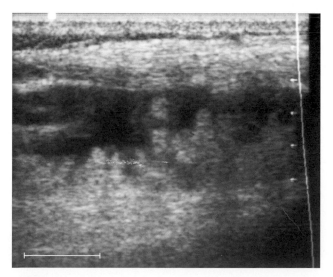 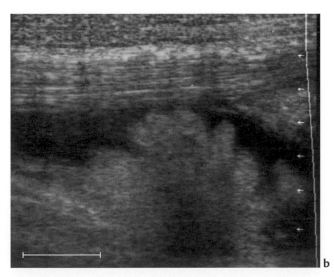

Fig. 90
Villous synovial thickening in a patient with rheumatoid arthritis (**a**). Villonodular synovitis was found in this patient's knee. The other joints were normal. Differential diagnosis includes PVNS, and infections such as tuberculosis, fungi, or Lyme disease (**b**).

Basic Signs of Pathology: Cartilage

Traumatic

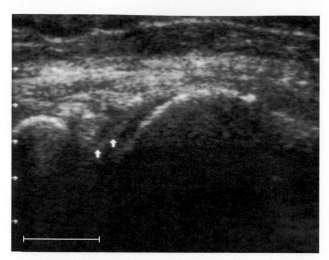

Fig. 91
A hypoechoic linear tear in the internal hyperechoic meniscus
(→).

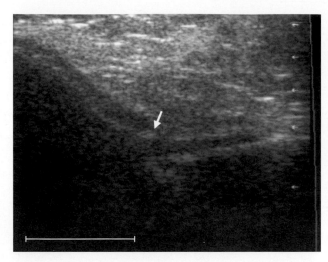

Fig. 92
An osteochondral fracture of the trochlea is seen as a hyperechoic focus (→) in the cartilage and an interruption of the cortical line.

Ultrasound is able to detect lesions in cartilage. Potential indications are peripheral meniscal tears in the knee joint, osteochondral fractures, and loose bodies. Meniscal tears are seen as a hypoechoic cleft in the hyperechoic meniscus. In articular cartilage, when accessible, ulcerations are seen as irregular thinning. Osteocartilaginous fractures appear as hyperechoic lines in the hypoechoic hyaline cartilage.

Degenerative

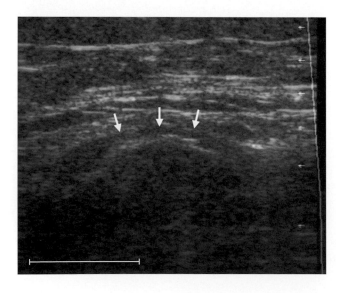

Fig. 93
Focal thinning of the hypoechoic cartilage on the medial condyle as a sign of degeneration (→).

Degenerative changes in the hyaline cartilage can also be evaluated when accessible to ultrasound. Focal thinning or ulcerations can be seen. The underlying subchondral bone is often irregular when degenerative changes are present.

Pathology

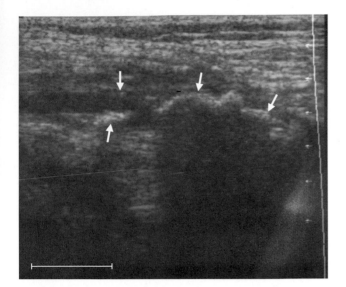

Fig. 94
Calcified atheromatous wall of the popliteal artery (→).

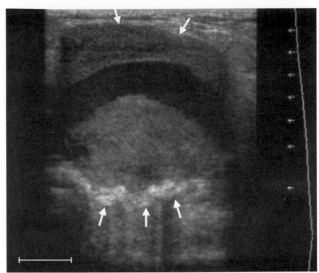

Fig. 95
Popliteal aneurysm (→) with a hyperechoic parietal thrombus and a calcified posterior wall.

Arterial pathology can be discovered when performing ultrasound of the soft tissues. Typical findings are calcified or occluded vessels, aneurysm, or pseudoaneurysm. In atherosclerosis, arterial walls are irregular and may be calcified. A frequent site of aneurysm is the popliteal artery. The aneurysms are bilateral in 30–50% of cases and often contain thrombi. Potential complications are rupture and distal emboli. Pseudo-aneurysms, mostly of traumatic origin, may also result from percutaneous puncture. Color Doppler demonstrates flow in the pseudo-aneurysm, differentiating it from a periarterial hematoma. Mycotic pseudoaneurysms are seen in bacterial endocarditis, but also in intravenous drug addicts. They have the same ultrasonographic characteristics as other aneurysms.

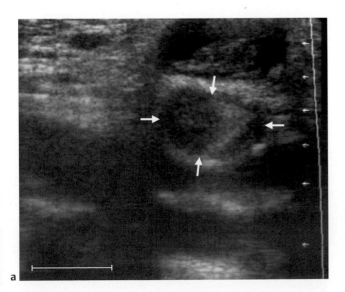
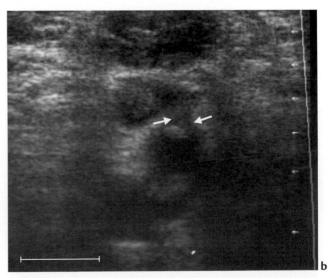

Fig. 96
A partially thrombosed pseudoaneurysm (→) arising from the anterior wall of the common femoral artery in a longitudinal scan (**a**). A transverse image shows the communication with the artery (→) (**b**).

Pathology

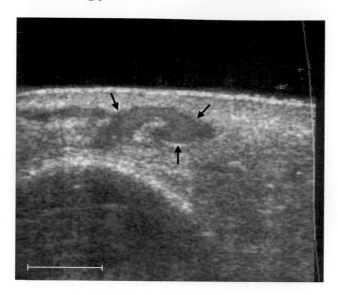

Fig. 97
Thrombophlebitis with hyperechoic material in the lumen of a superficial varicosity (→) in front of the tibia in this case of erysipelas.

Venous pathology, such as varices and thrombophlebitis, should be recognized when performing musculoskeletal ultrasound. In deep venous thrombosis, ultrasound shows echoic material within the venous lumen, which is not compressible. Ultrasound can also show thrombosis in superficial veins, frequently seen in the lower extremity, with the same characteristics. Varicosities are shown as a network of anechoic bands in the subcutaneous tissue.

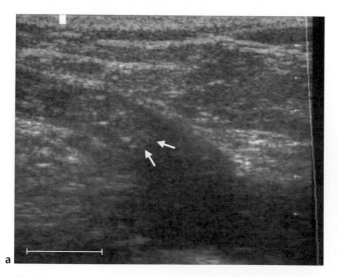

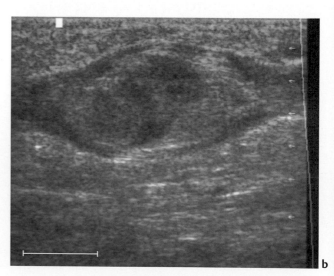

Fig. 98
Fresh thrombus is seen in the great saphenous vein with its rounded tip (→) at the entrance of the femoral vein (**a**). A longitudinal scan of the great saphenous vein 10 cm more caudally shows a large, heterogeneous echoic thrombus (**b**).

Inflammation

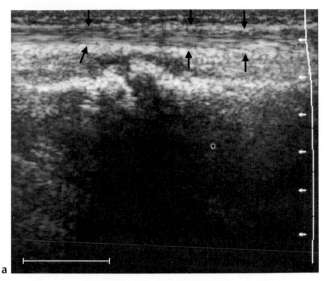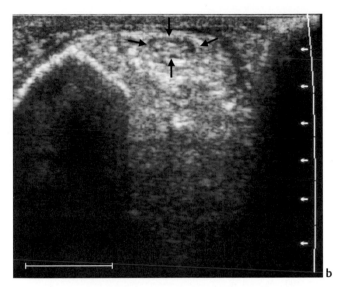

Fig. 99
This patient presented with a stress fracture of the proximal fibula. The overlying peroneal nerve has a hypoechoic appearence (→) especially at the periphery, on longitudinal (**a**) and transverse (**b**) scans, typical of neuritis.

In neuritis, the nerve appears thickened and hypoechoic, particularly at the periphery of the cross section. Neuritis often results form continuous compression or contusion. A special form of neuritis is entrapment, as in carpal tunnel syndrome (see Wrist, below).

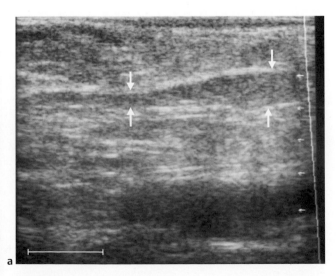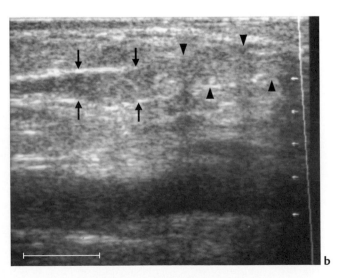

Fig. 100
Longitudinal scans of the femoral nerve show a thickened hypoechoic aspect (→), due to scar tissue (▶) after previous surgery in the groin (**a** and **b**).

Neurinoma and Neurofibroma

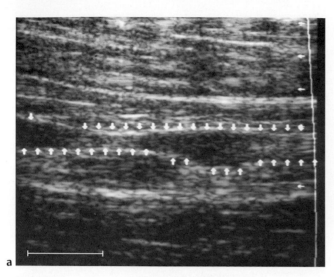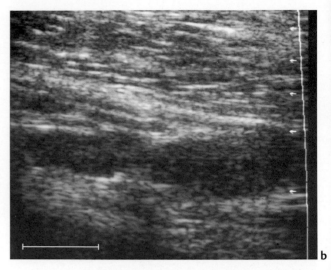

Fig. 101
Longitudinal scans of the sciatic nerve show hypoechoic ovoid neurofibromatous lesions anterior to the gluteus maximus muscle (→)(**a**) and between the biceps and adductor magnus muscle (**b**). Only small portions of the normal hyperechoic nerve are seen.

These benign tumors are usually fusiform, parallel to the long axis of the nerve. Neurinoma appears as a hypoechoic and well defined elongated or ovoid mass. Many soft-tissue tumors appear hypoechoic, but the localization along the course of a nerve allows specific diagnosis. Hypoechoic neuroma can also develop in scar tissue.

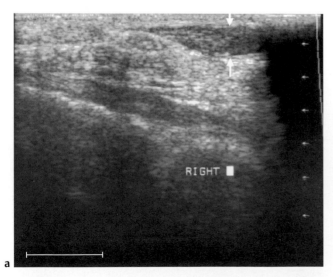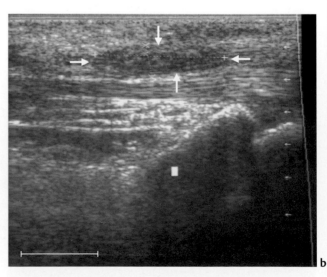

Fig. 102
A hypoechoic neurinoma is seen in a transverse (→) (**a**) and longitudinal (→) scan (**b**) in the hypodermis after reparative surgery for a sectioned palmaris longus tendon.

Fracture

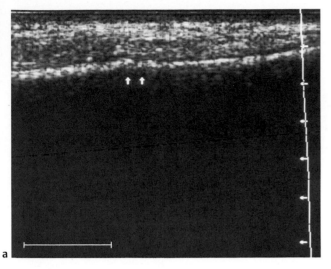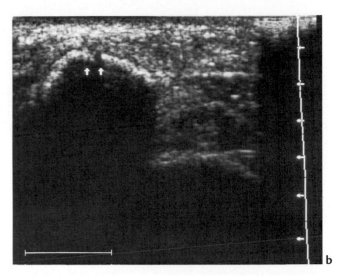

Fig. 103
A longitudinal (**a**) and an axial (**b**) scan of the distal fibula show cortical interruption (→) diagnostic for a small fracture.

Small fractures or bone avulsions can be found on an ultrasound examination, when the examination is guided by the symptoms and clinical evaluation of the patient. A fracture appears as a discontinuity in the highly reflecting bone–soft-tissue interface. Fractures can also be detected by recognizing subperiosteal hemorrhage, which is hypoechoic and elevates the normal hyperechoic periosteum. Ultrasound is useful in the detection of bone impactions, such as Hill–Sachs lesions, which appear as a defect of the postero-lateral contour of the humeral head.

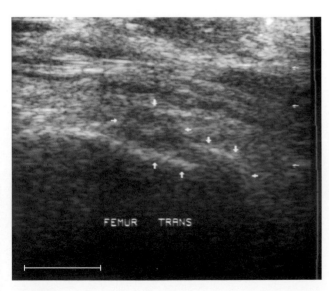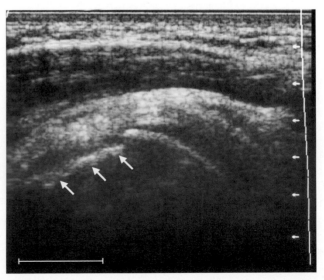

Fig. 104
A larger recent fracture of the anterior cortex of the femur with an oblique sagittal course on the plain film, seen as a cortical interruption and an adjacent hematoma (→) on this axial image.

Fig. 105
An impaction on the postero-lateral surface of the humeral head or Hill–Sachs lesion (→) secondary to an antero-inferior luxation of the shoulder.

Stress Fracture

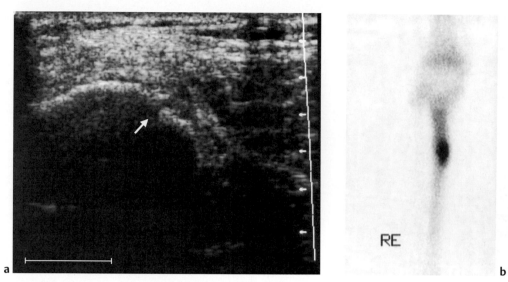

Fig. 106
A stress fracture at the anteromedial cortex of the proximal tibia (→) (**a**). Positive nuclear bone scan (**b**).

Stress fractures are easily detected by ultrasound (see also the section on the foot, p. 176 ff). The periosteal reaction presents as a hyperechoic line elevated by a hy-poechoic callus overlying the cortical interruption (see also callus formation, p. 50).

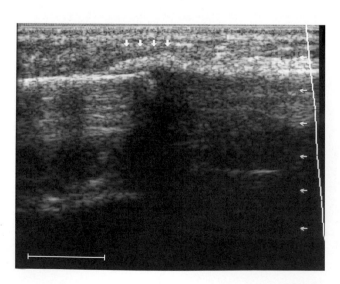

Fig. 107
A long-standing stress fracture shows a thickened mature periosteal reaction (→) covering and obliterating the fracture site.

Osteomyelitis

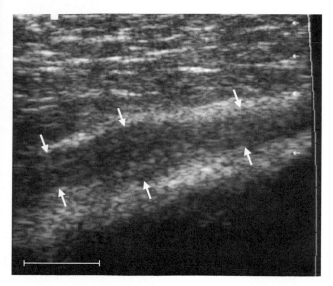

Fig. 108
A hypoechoic collection (→) is noted between the hyperechoic periosteum and the cortex in a case of acute osteomyelitis.

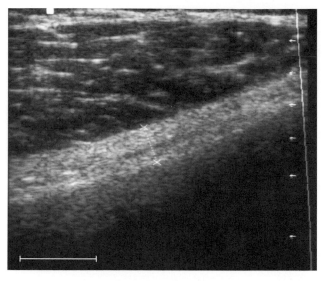

Fig. 109
Sagittal view of the distal femur: mature periosteal reaction due to chronic osteomyelitis.

In acute osteomyelitis, a subperiosteal collection can be observed as a hypoechoic zone surrounding the cortical bone, bordered by a hyperechoic line. In chronic osteomyelitis, a mature periosteal reaction appears as a thickened hyperechoic periosteal band. A reactivation of chronic osteomyelitis is demonstrated by the presence of subperiosteal fluid and/or soft-tissue abscesses.

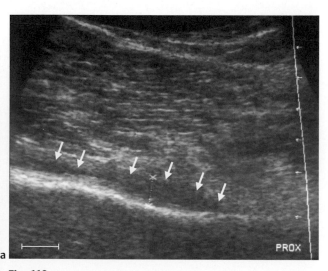

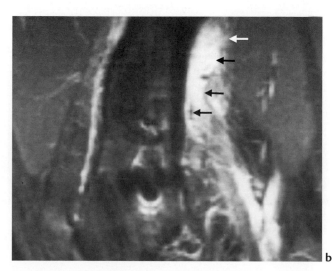

Fig. 110
A posterior longitudinal view of the distal femur: mixed periosteal reaction, suggesting reactivation in a patient with chronic osteomyelitis of the femur (→) (**a**). MRI of the same patient (fat-saturated T_1-weighted gadolinium-enhanced image): the collections are well seen at the bony surface (→) (**b**).

Basic Signs of Pathology: Evaluation of Orthopaedic Procedures

Callus Formation

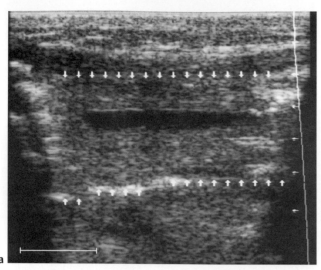
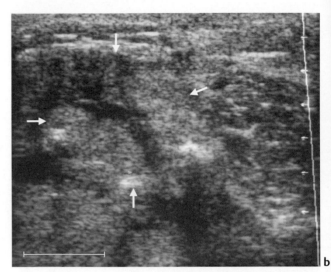

Fig. 111
Ultrasound evaluation of an Ilizarov leg-lengthening procedure shows homogeneous callus formation (→) with calcifications at the periphery and a central fluid-filled cavity in these longitudinal (**a**) and axial (**b**) scans.

Ultrasound is useful to evaluate early bone production at the distraction site of the Ilizarov procedure. The detection of new bone formation determines the choice of the rate of distraction, and is possible by ultrasound many weeks before radiography becomes positive. Callus formation appears as echoic foci at the distraction site, aligned in the longitudinal plane and increasing in volume over time. Cysts located in the callus can also be detected and aspirated if they persist.

Infection

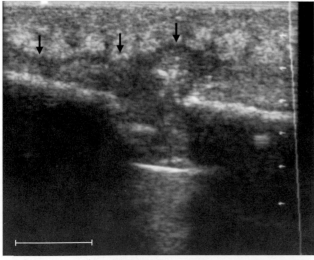
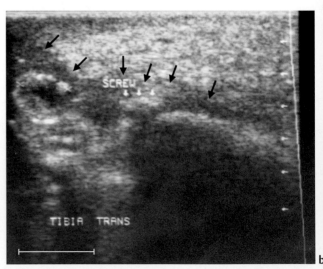

Fig. 112
Infected plates and screws appear as hyperechoic structures; a hypoechoic, bandlike collection (→) elevates the periosteum and surrounds the screws (**a** and **b**).

Ultrasound is able to detect signs of infection, such as periosteal reaction or soft tissue collections, particularly in the presence of metallic devices. Other imaging modalities such as MRI or CT are inefficient due to image degradation by artifacts.

Prostheses

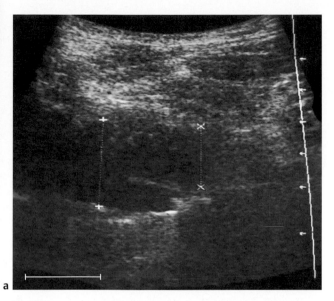
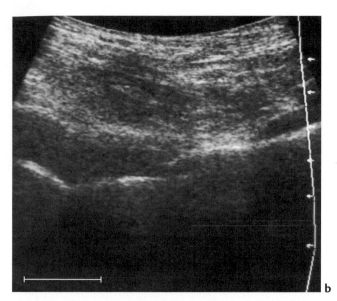

Fig. 113
Infected hip prosthesis: elevation of the pseudocapsule on the longitudinal scan (**a**). Normal sized pseudocapsule (**b**).

The major complications of hip prostheses are mechanical loosening of the prosthesis and infection, which are clinically and radiographically similar. On ultrasound, the most specific sign of infection is the presence of extra-articular fluid cavities or abscesses. Another sign is a distension of the pseudocapsule at the prosthetic-diaphyseal junction. Ultrasound is useful to evaluate the dislocation of a radiolucent prosthesis component, such as silicone.

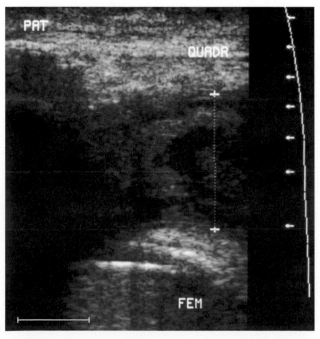

Fig. 114
A heterogeneous collection located between the quadriceps tendon and the femoral component in a total knee prosthesis.

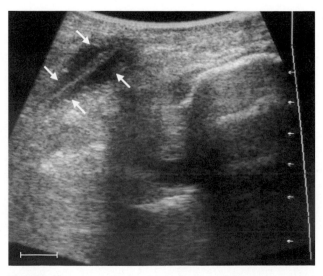

Fig. 115
Displaced component of a total knee prosthesis, which had migrated in a suprapatellar location (→), seen here on a sagittal scan.

Basic Signs of Pathology: Skin

Scar

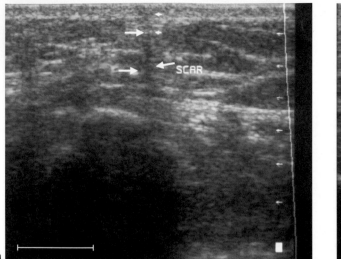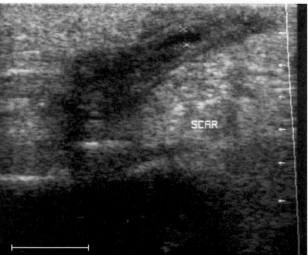

Fig. 116
A typical image of a scar is a hyperechoic focus with a posterior shadow (→) (**a**). This infected scar is thickened, hypoechoic, poorly delimited, and contains a fluid collection (**b**).

A scar can have various appearances, but most frequently shows as a hyperechoic zone in the relatively hypoechoic subcutaneous tissue. It can contain calcifications. When infected, the scar is thick, hypoechoic, and may contain small residual collections. A fistulous sinus tract appears as an irregular hypoechoic or anechoic channel.

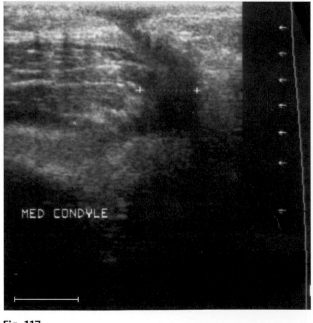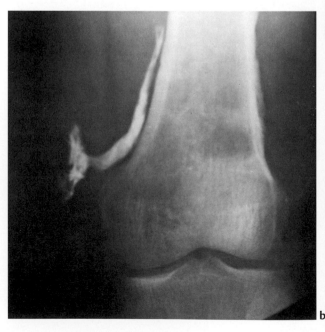

Fig. 117
This fistulous track is well evaluated with ultrasound, as shown in a coronal scan in a patient with chronic osteomyelitis (**a**). Fistulography for comparison (**b**).

Edema

Fig. 118
Diffuse thickening and hyperechogenicity of both the skin and the subcutaneous fat, which become indistinct, shown in a patient with erysipelas, on a comparative study (**a** and **b**).

The most frequent pathological change in the subcutaneous tissue is edema. The subcutaneous tissue is thickened and hyperechoic, with an inversion of the normal appearance. When edematous changes have occurred, fibrous septae become hypoechoic, and the surrounding fat hyperechoic. Edema can be caused by various pathologies: cellulitis, venous insufficiency, lymphedema. Lymphoma is a differential diagnosis. When edema increases, lamellar fluid collections can be found.

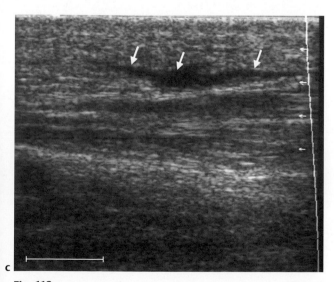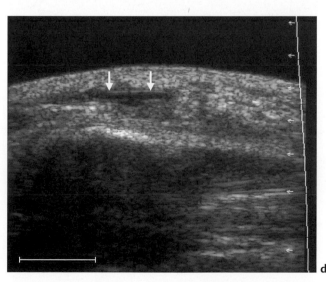

Fig. 118
In extensive edema, as in lymphedema (**c**) or algoneurodystrophy (**d**), small pools of fluid (→) dissect the subcutaneous fat.

Basic Signs of Pathology: Skin

Lipoma

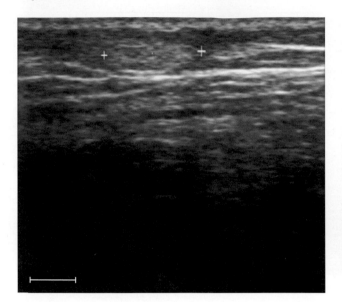

Fig. 119
A hyperechoic lipoma in front of the triceps muscle.

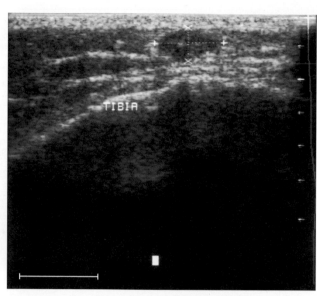

Fig. 120
A hypoechoic lipoma near the anterior tibial cortex with fascial adherence is seen. This lipoma could not be mobilized.

Lipomas can have variable echogenicity. The diagnosis is best established by density measurements on CT. Ultrasound, however, can determine the relationship with the surrounding structures and demonstrate the mobility of the lesion. Completely mobile small lipomas can be enucleated by local excision.

Echogenicity depends on the proportion of fat and water content in the lipoma. The most frequent presentation is an elongated mass, which is isoechoic or hyperechoic to the surrounding fat. Hypoechoic lipomas should be differentiated from subcutaneous lymphadenopathy, which has a typical bean shape.

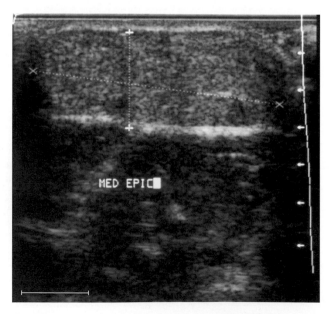

Fig. 121
A hyperechoic subcutaneous lipoma is in contact with the bony surface of the medial epicondyle of the elbow.

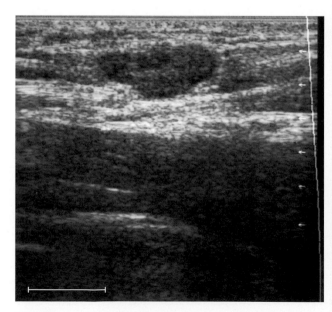

Fig. 122
A tender, inflamed subcutaneous lymph node in the groin.

Cyst

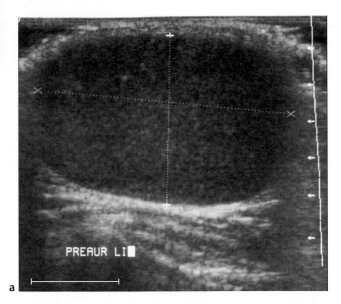 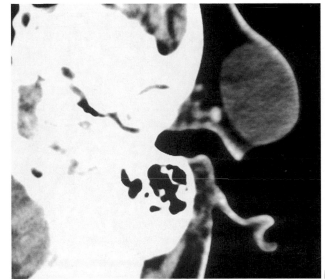

Fig. 123
A homogeneous hypoechoic epidermoid cyst is found in the preauricular subcutis (**a**). Corresponding CT (**b**).

Cyst-like structures of various etiologies can be encountered in the subcutaneous fat. Epidermoid sebaceous cysts are frequently found, and present as homogeneous hypoechoic masses. Liponecrosis can become encapsulated, and presents as a hypoechoic mass, which can contain calcifications and is surrounded by a hyperechoic wall. It may resemble chronic bursitis.

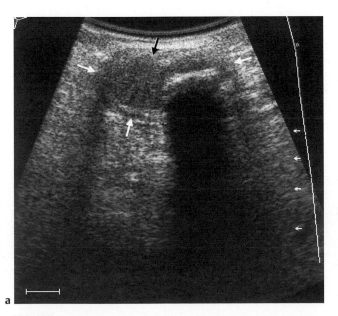 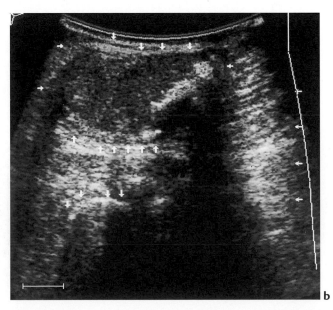

Fig. 124
An encapsulated liponecrosis (→) with a hypoechoic content and calcifications delimited by a hyperechoic wall in front of the greater trochanter (**a** and **b**).

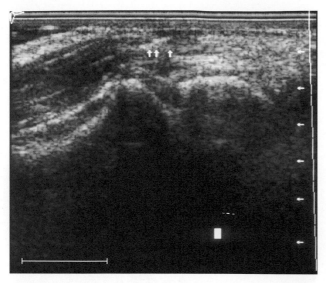

Fig. 125
Ultrasound detects a small wooden splinter (→) and shows its extra-articular localization in front of the metacarpo-phalangeal joint of the thumb.

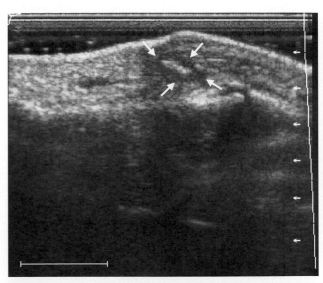

Fig. 126
Hypoechoic granulation tissue surrounds this foreign body (→) in front of the distal part of P1 of the second finger on a posterior sagittal scan.

Unrecognized foreign bodies can lead to complications, such as infection or erosion into vessels. Plain radiographs only detect foreign bodies usually consisting of metal or glass. Ultrasound is useful in the detection and localization of radiolucent foreign bodies such as wood or thorns. Pieces of wood are best visualized, followed by glass, plastic, and metal. Pieces of wood are initially hyperechoic, with possible acoustic shadowing. They are often surrounded by an inflammatory reaction, which appears hypoechoic, and is responsible for the progressive decomposition of the wood, which becomes less echoic and finally can even disappear.

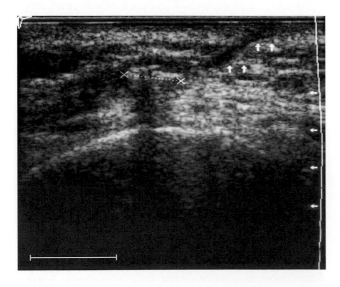

Fig. 127
A disintegrated wooden foreign body in front of the proximal tibia. The cutaneous entrance is visible (→).

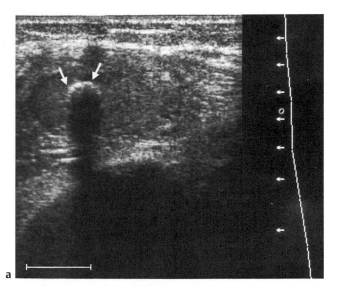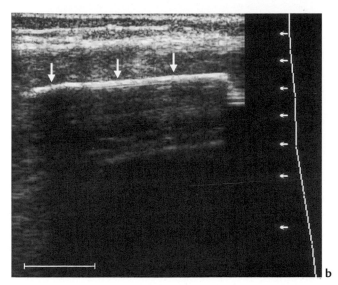

Fig. 128
In this patient, a piece of wood was visualized in the vastus medialis muscle as a hyperechoic line (→) causing a posterior shadow, surrounded by a large collection of pus, illustrated in axial (**a**) and sagittal (**b**) planes.

Plastic foreign bodies are slightly less echoic than wood, and can also create an acoustic shadow. Glass and metal produce strong, significant reverberation artifacts, also called comet's tail artifact. This artifact helps to identify the nature of the foreign body. Measurements and localization are still possible. Secondary signs associated with foreign bodies are: hematoma, purulent or inflammatory reaction, and in the acute phase, air, shown as echoic foci with a dirty shadow. Even when a radiopaque foreign body is seen on radiography, ultrasound is still indicated for optimal localization and detection of local complications.

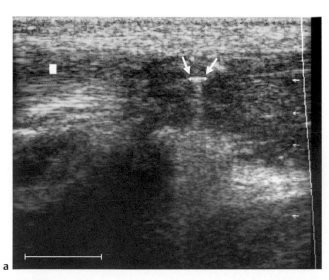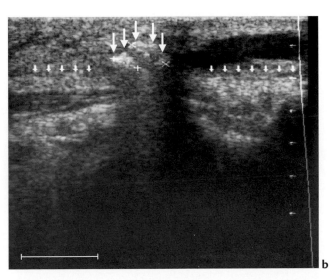

Fig. 129
In this patient, glass fragments were visible on a plain film at the level of the lateral epicondyle. Ultrasound showed these fragments with their typical artifacts (→), located in the extensor carpi radialis muscles (**a**). An associated fluid collection proximal to the fragments was detected (**b**).

Puncture

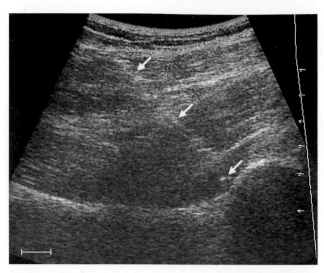

Fig. 130
Ultrasound-guided diagnostic aspiration of septic arthritis shows the hyperechoic needle (→).

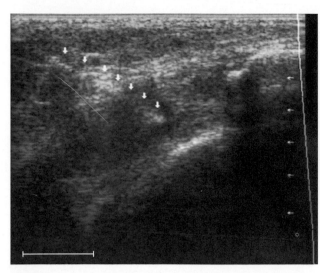

Fig. 131
Puncture and infiltration of a hypoechoic pannus in the knee joint of a patient with rheumatoid arthritis (→).

When puncture is mandatory for treatment or to determine the appropriate management, ultrasound offers real-time guidance. Puncture can be used for cytology or histology in tumors; in aspiration and drainage in infectious or inflammatory disorders; or for guided injection of drugs in focal inflammatory conditions (pannus formation, bursitis). Specially designed probes or probe adaptors, needles with echoic markers, and other modalities can be helpful in ultrasound-guided puncture.

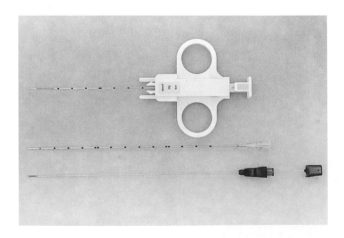

Fig. 132
Examples of needles marked at their tip or at fixed intervals.

Normal and Pathologic Regional Ultrasound Upper Extremities

Shoulder

Upper Arm

Elbow

Forearm

Wrist

Hand

Shoulder

Anatomy

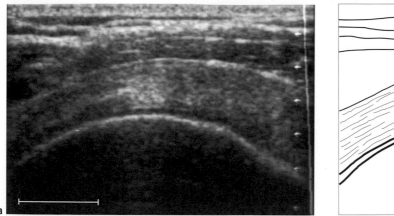

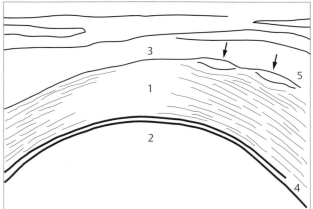

Fig. 133
Transverse scan of the supraspinatus tendon (**1**), humeral head (**2**), deltoid muscle (**3**), cartilage (**4**), subdeltoid bursa (→) (**5**) (**a** and **b**).

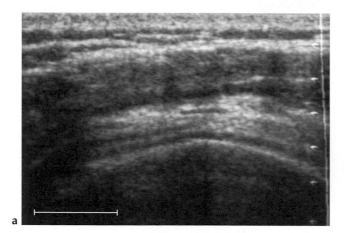

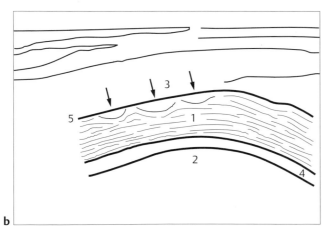

Fig. 134
Transverse scan of the infraspinatus tendon (**1**), humeral head (**2**), deltoid muscle (**3**), cartilage (**4**), subdeltoid bursa (→) (**5**) (**a** and **b**).

Fig. 135
Position for rotator cuff evaluation in a transverse plane.

The shoulder is scanned in internal rotation and hyperextension with the patient seated. This position allows the cuff to rotate anteriorly from underneath the acromion and also to accentuate small tears by increasing stress on the tendons. The tendons are imaged in a transverse and coronal plane. Different layers of the shoulder are routinely identified. The skin and hypoechoic subcutaneous fat are located most superficially; the deltoid muscle forms the next layer and is less echoic than the underlying tendons.

Anatomy

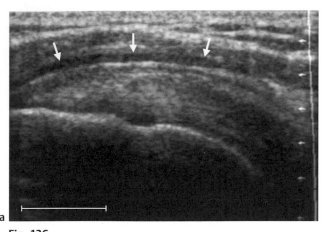
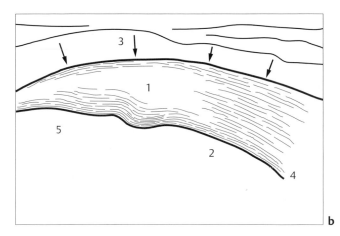

Fig. 136
Coronal scan of the supraspinatus tendon (**1**), humeral head (**2**), deltoid muscle (**3**), cartilage (**4**), subdeltoid bursa (→), greater tuberosity (**5**) (**a** and **b**).

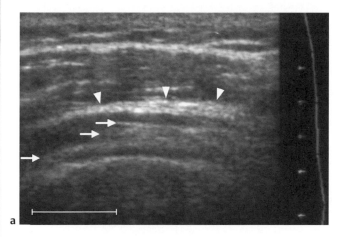

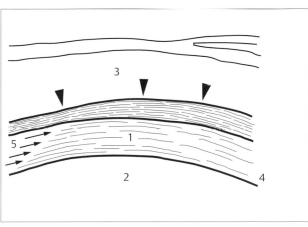

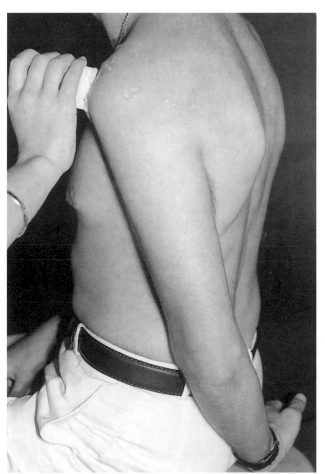

Fig. 137
Coronal scan of the infraspinatus tendon (**1**), humeral head (**2**), deltoid muscle (**3**), cartilage (**4**), subdeltoid bursa (▶), musculotendinous junction (→) (**5**) (**a** and **b**).

Fig. 138
Position for rotator cuff evaluation in a coronal plane.

There is a thin hyperechoic plane located deep in the deltoid muscle formed by the subdeltoid bursa and the surrounding fat. The supra- and infraspinatus tendons, which are part of the rotator cuff, form the next layer and appear hyperechoic. The hypoechoic hyaline cartilage on the humeral head is the layer beneath the rotator cuff.

Shoulder

Anatomy

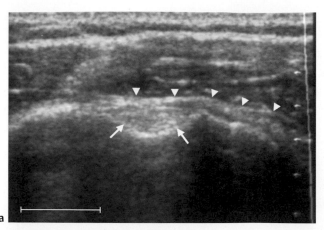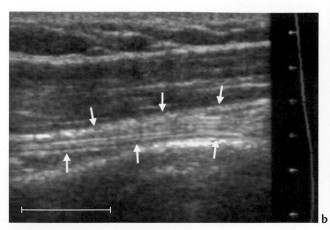

Fig. 139
Biceps tendon (→) on transverse (**a**) and on longitudinal scans (**b**). Transverse ligament (**a**) (▶), deltoid muscle seen above the biceps tendon (**a** and **b**).

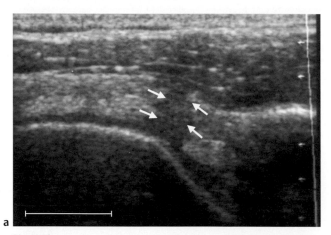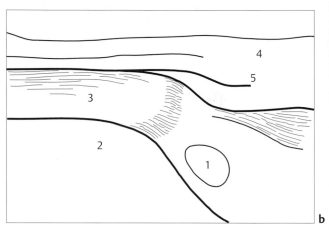

Fig. 140
The rotator cuff interval corresponds to the space between the anterior aspect of the supraspinatus tendon and the long biceps tendon. It is seen on a transverse scan as a hypoechoic zone (→). Biceps tendon (**1**), humeral head (**2**), rotator cuff (**3**), deltoid muscle (**4**), subdeltoid bursa (**5**) (**a** and **b**).

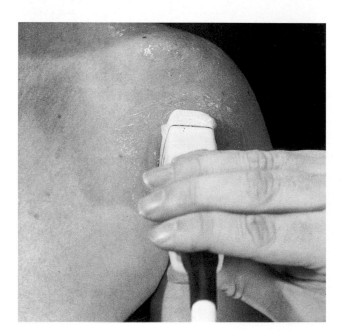

The biceps tendon is examined in a transverse and longitudinal plane. It should be seen within the biceps tendon groove as an echoic circle or ellipse on the transverse plane and as an echoic fibrillar band on a longitudinal view. On a transverse scan, the acromion can be seen medially to the long biceps tendon. The hypoechoic rotator cuff interval is seen between the biceps tendon and the rotator cuff. The biceps tendon is surrounded by a synovial sheath, that commmunicates with the glenohumeral joint. Anteriorly, the tendon is covered by the transverse ligament, the subdeltoid bursa, and the deltoid muscle.

Fig. 141
Position for evaluation of the biceps tendon.

Anatomy

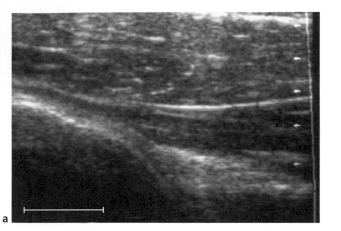
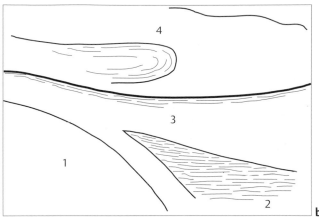

Fig. 142
Transverse scan of the posterior labrum shown by a posterior approach. Humeral head (**1**), posterior labrum (**2**), infraspinatus (**3**), deltoid muscle (**4**) (**a** and **b**).

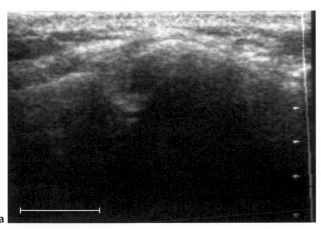
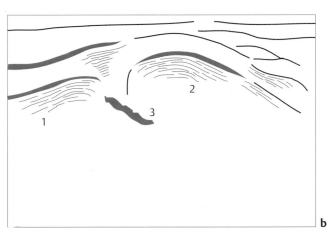

Fig. 143
Acromioclavicular joint on a coronal scan. Acromion (**1**), clavicle (**2**), meniscus (**3**) (**a** and **b**).

The normal triangular hyperechoic posterior labrum can be examined routinely on a transverse scan by a posterior approach. The posterior labrum is covered by a millimetric anechoic posterior articular recess and the infraspinatus muscle. By rotating the arm externally, the subscapularis tendon is brought parallel to the probe and visualized in its long axis in a transverse anterior approach. This maneuver also fills the posterior articular recess.

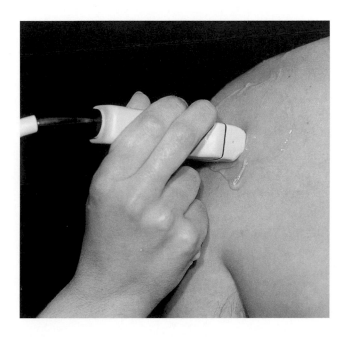

Fig. 144
Position for the evaluation of the posterior labrum.

Anatomy

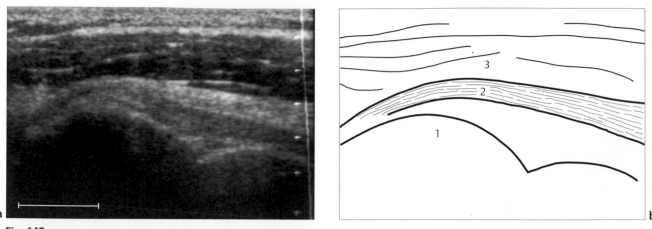

Fig. 145
Subscapularis tendon shown on a transverse scan by an anterior approach. Lesser tuberosity of the humerus (**1**), subscapularis tendon (**2**), deltoid muscle (**3**) (**a** and **b**).

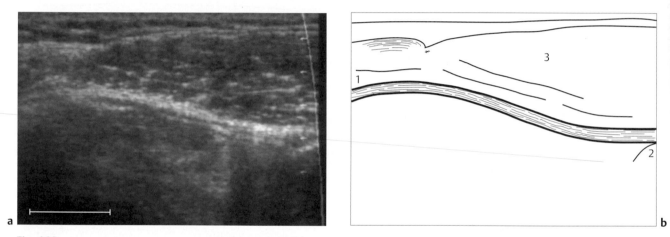

Fig. 146
Transverse scan of the coracoacromial ligament (**1**), coracoid process (**2**), deltoid muscle (**3**) (**a** and **b**).

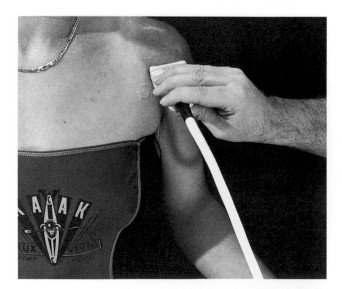

Fig. 147
Position for the evaluation of the subscapularis tendon.

Potential pitfalls of normal anatomy should be recognized, since they can be misdiagnosed as tears. They include muscle bundles penetrating the cuff (frequently present in the infraspinatus tendon), acoustic shadowing arising from fibrous septae in the subcutaneous fat or deltoid muscle, hypoechoic tendon insertion, rotator cuff interval, and oblique scanning responsible for a hypoechoic tendon appearance (see artifacts).

Rotator Cuff: Full-Thickness Tear

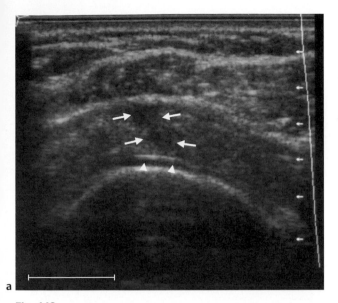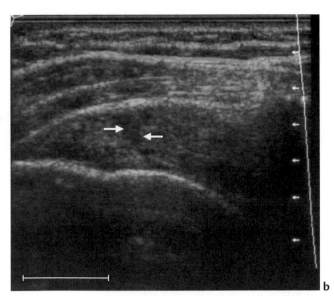

Fig. 148
A small full-thickness tear is seen in the supraspinatus tendon as an anechoic cleft (→) in the transverse (**a**) and coronal planes (**b**). Note the cartilage interface sign (▶).

The signs associated with full-thickness tear are: complete absence of the cuff, hypoechoic or anechoic cleft in the cuff, direct joint communication through a tendon gap with a distended subacromial-subdeltoid bursa, naked tuberosity (focal apposition of deltoid muscle on greater tuberosity), focal cartilage interface sign (focal hyperechogenicity of humeral head cartilage due to enhancement posterior to an anechoic cleft), focal atrophy, and hernia of the deltoid muscle or of the subacromial-subdeltoid bursa in the cuff.

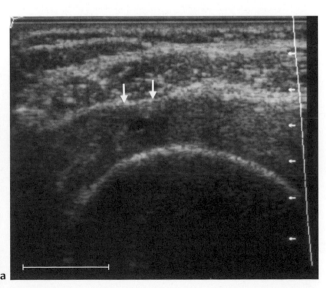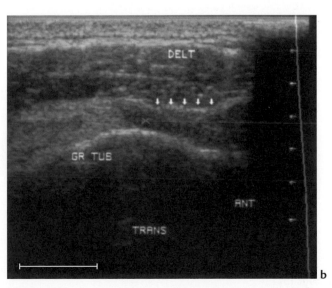

Fig. 149
Two examples of herniation (→) of the deltoid muscle, indicating a full-thickness tear (**a** and **b**).

Shoulder

Rotator Cuff: Full-Thickness Tear

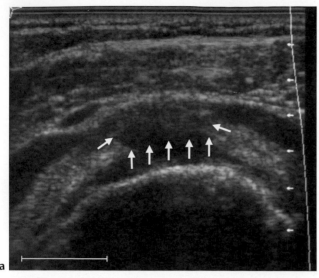

a

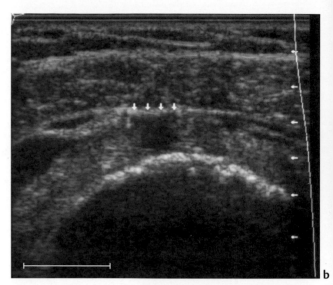

b

Fig. 150
Direct communication through a tendon gap (→) with a distended subacromiodeltoid bursa as a direct sign of a full-thickness tear seen in two transverse scans (**a** and **b**).

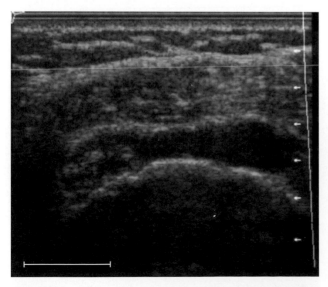

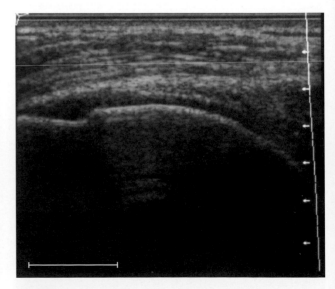

Fig. 151
No cuff was found under a fluid-filled subdeltoid bursa in this transverse scan.

Fig. 152
A naked tuberosity seen on a coronal scan is good proof of a full-thickness tear.

Rotator Cuff: Full-Thickness Tear

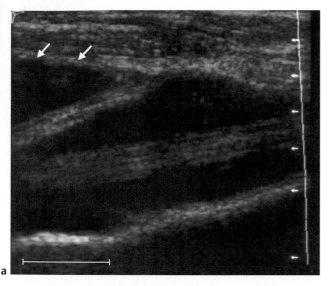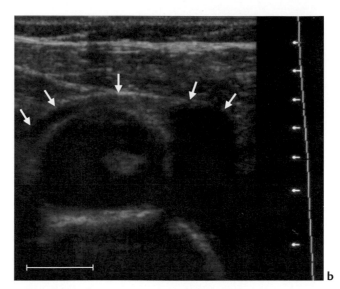

Fig. 153
A large effusion in the biceps tendon sheath is present, accompanying a full-thickness tear, shown in longitudinal (**a**) and transverse planes (**b**). The fluid-filled subdeltoid bursa (→) covers the tendon sheath.

Secondary signs associated with rupture of the rotator cuff are : gleno-humeral joint effusion, subacromial-subdeltoid bursitis, effusion in the biceps tendon sheath, and acromio-clavicular effusion (Geiser sign). This sign is only seen when there is communication between the subacromial-subdeltoid bursa and the acromioclavicular joint, allowing fluid to extend from the glenohumeral joint. Another secondary sign is surface irregularity of the greater tuberosity, often associated with impingement syndrome.

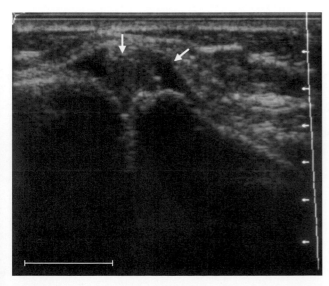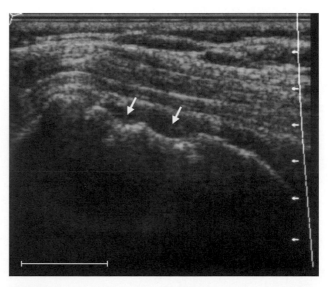

Fig. 154
Effusion of the acromioclavicular joint (→), also called the Geiser sign.

Fig. 155
Surface irregularities (→) of the greater tuberosity are seen in this patient with a full-thickness tear.

Shoulder

Rotator Cuff: Partial-Thickness- and Intrasubstance Tears

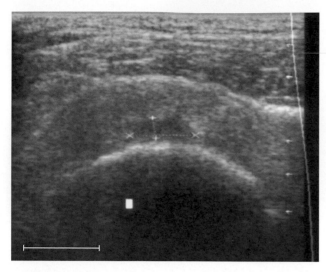

Fig. 156
A partial-thickness tear is measured at the under surface of the cuff on a transverse scan.

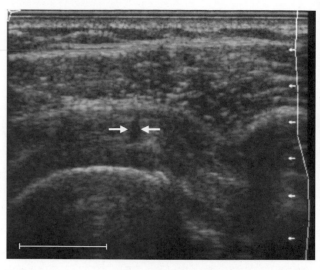

Fig. 157
A partial-thickness tear (→) at the upper surface of the rotator cuff is shown in the anterior part of the supraspinatus tendon 3 mm from the rotator cuff interval.

Partial-thickness tears of the rotator cuff appear as an anechoic or hypoechoic cleft in the cuff, which can be situated on the undersurface of the cuff (and seen on an arthrogram), within the substance of the cuff, or on the upper surface of the cuff (neither seen on an arthrogram). Their borders tend to be hyperechoic in comparison to the adjacent tendons. They are often associated with subacromial-subdeltoid bursitis.

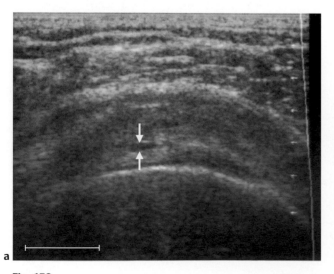

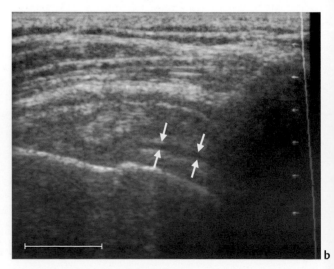

Fig. 158
A small, anechoic intrasubstance tear (→) in the supraspinatus tendon, in axial (**a**) and coronal (**b**) planes.

Impingement Syndrome

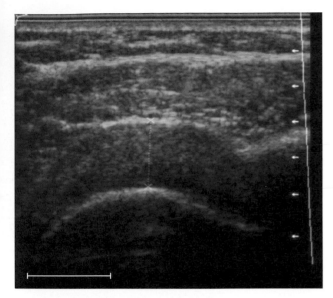

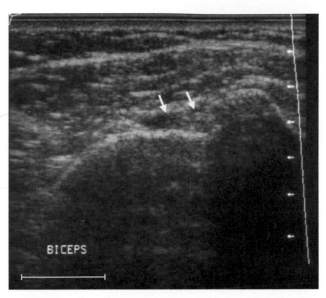

Fig. 159
In this patient, the rotator cuff is diffusely hypoechoic and appears swollen (more than 2 mm) in comparison to the other side: impingement syndrome, stage I.

Fig. 160
A small amount of fluid (→) surrounds the otherwise normal biceps tendon in this patient, who clinically suffered from impingement syndrome.

Impingement syndrome is caused by chronic entrapment of the rotator cuff and the subacromial bursa between the humeral head and the acromion. This entity has been classified in three stages by Neer: stage I corresponds to edema and hemorrhage in the bursa and the rotator cuff; stage II to fibrosis, thickening of subacromial soft tissue, and sometimes to partial rupture of the rotator cuff; in stage III there is complete rupture of the rotator cuff. Stages II and III have already been discussed under partial and full thickness rotator cuff tears. In stages I and II, the most reliable sign is fluid in the subacromial subdeltoid bursa. An additional sign is a difference of more than 2 mm in the thickness of the rotator cuff in comparison with the contralateral side.

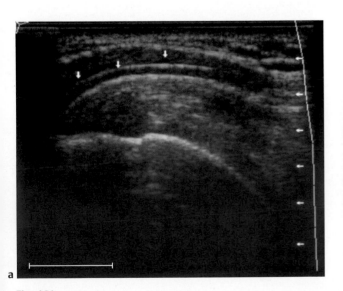

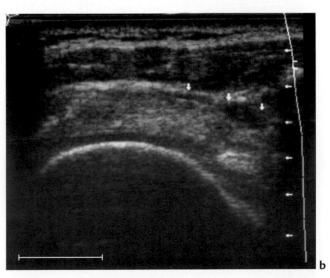

a

b

Fig. 161
Subacromial-subdeltoid fluid-filled bursitis (→) in a coronal plane, together with a thick hypoechoic rotator cuff in this case of impingement syndrome (**a**). On a transverse scan, a small bursitis (→) can be seen that accumulates in front of the rotator cuff interval (**b**).

Shoulder

Impingement Syndrome

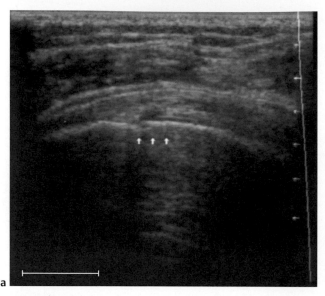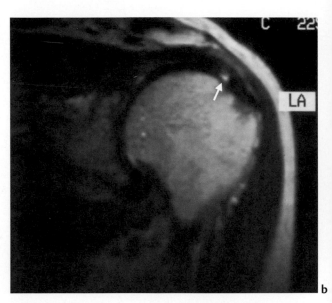

Fig. 162
Marked thinning and a small partial-thickness tear (→) shown as a hypoechoic zone, is part of a stage II impingement syndrome (**a**). The MRI of the same patient gives a hyperintense signal on a T_2-weighted image, corresponding to the partial tear (→) (**b**).

A small effusion in the biceps tendon sheath can also be a sign of impingement of the rotator cuff. Subacromial-subdeltoid bursitis associated with impingement syndrome is not always anechoic, but can present with a thickened wall and echoic contents, without fluid. Bursitis has to be looked for where fluid can accumulate, at the outer or anterior aspect of the shoulder, and not below the acromion process. In the impingement syndrome, a thickened bursa can accumulate in front of the acromion when the arm is abducted or elevated, instead of gliding under the acromion together with the rotator cuff tendons.

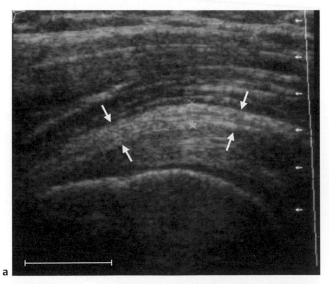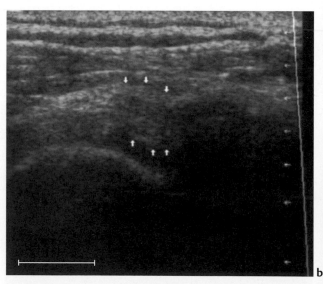

Fig. 163
Hyperechoic thickened bursa (→) (**a**). During abduction of the arm, the thickened bursa accumulates at the outer border of the acromion and forms a hyperechoic nodule (→) (**b**).

Calcified Tendinitis

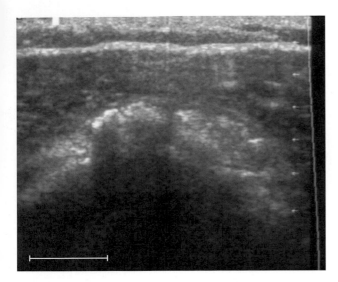

Fig. 164
Hyperechoic foci with a posterior acoustic shadow are found in the infraspinatus tendon at its insertion, corresponding to calcified deposits.

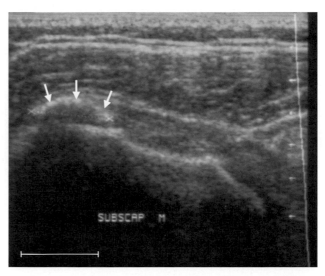

Fig. 165
An arciform calcification without a shadow (→) is shown at the insertion of the subscapular tendon on the lesser tuberosity, not visible on plain films.

Calcifications are seen as hyperechoic foci with or without acoustic shadow. It is important to look at plain films before the ultrasound examination, because calcifications can produce a false image of rupture.

Calcifications are almost never associated with rotator cuff rupture. Ultrasound is an appropriate method of detecting calcifications in the subscapular tendon.

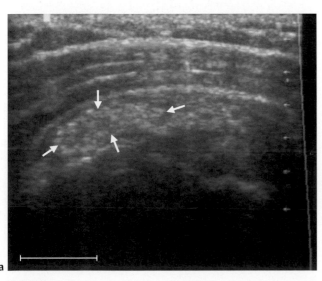

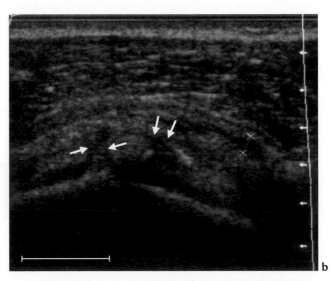

Fig. 166
This hyperechoic nodule (→) seen in the distal part of the supraspinatus tendon proved to be an amorphous deposit of calcium on the plain films (**a**). The calcifications within this rotator cuff cause shadows that mimic a tear (→). Notice also the small subdeltoideal bursitis (**b**).

Shoulder

Biceps Tendinitis

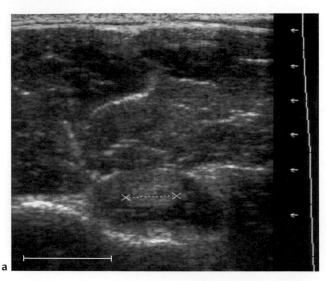
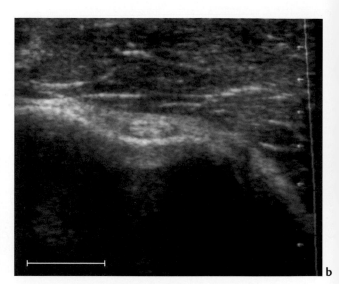

Fig. 167
A tender, thickened biceps tendon and a tendon sheath effusion are noted in this patient with tendinitis. No rotator cuff abnormality is seen (**a**). The normal opposite side is shown for comparison (**b**).

An effusion in the biceps tendon sheath can be seen in various situations, and is associated in 90% of cases with pathology elsewhere in the joint. In biceps ten-dinitis, effusion in the sheath is associated with focal tenderness and occasionally with heterogeneity of the tendon.

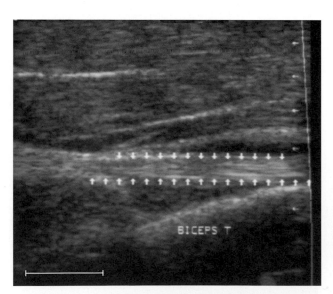
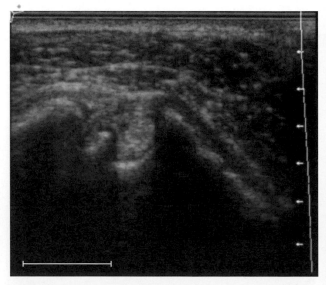

Fig. 168
Small sheath effusions are only seen at the proximal musculo-tendinous junction (→), as shown here in a sagittal plane.

Fig. 169
Degenerative changes in the bicipital groove create an irregular hyperechoic bone surface.

Biceps Tendon Rupture

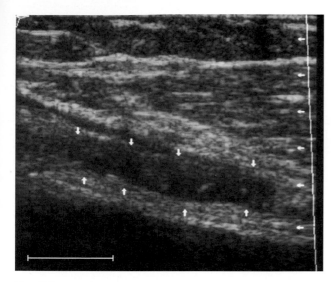

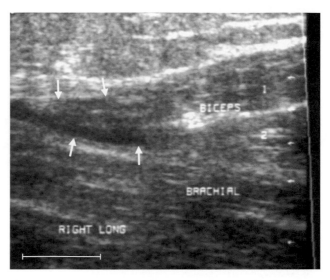

Fig. 170
An almost anechoic gap (→) is seen between the two ends of the tendon at the site of rupture.

Fig. 171
Another case of rupture is seen at the musculotendinous junction (→) where the muscle fibers end in a hypoechoic collection.

An empty bicipital groove can be caused by biceps tendon rupture or luxation. In case of rupture, the tendon is not visualized, and the groove is empty. On longitudinal scans, the retracted distal end of the tendon can be found.

Biceps Tendon Luxation

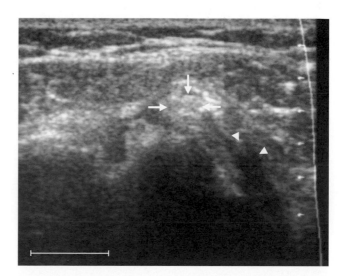

Fig. 172
The biceps tendon (→) is located medial to the lesser tuberosity and is associated with a rupture at the insertion of the subscapular tendon producing an anechoic gap (▶).

Biceps tendon luxation is often associated with rupture of the subscapular tendon. The transverse ligament, which is an expansion of this tendon, is torn. The dislocated tendon should be looked for in a medial position.

Shoulder

Effusion

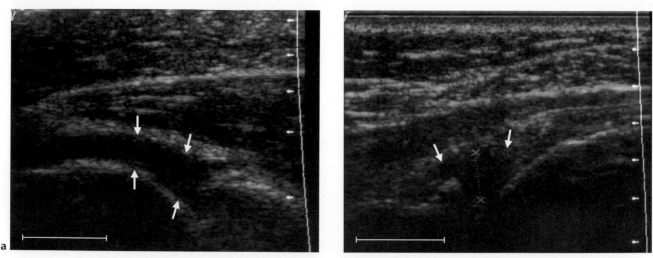

Fig. 173
Two examples of glenohumeral effusion presenting as an anechoic fluid collection (→) between the anterior aspect of the infraspinatus muscle and the glenohumeral joint (**a** and **b**).

The amount of effusion in the gleno-humeral joint is estimated by measuring the size of the posterior synovial recess, which is normally less than 2 mm. A posterior transverse scan at the middle of the gleno-humeral joint will show the infraspinatus tendon covering the glenoid labrum. Biceps tendon sheath effusion is also a sign of joint effusion. Glenohumeral effusion is a sign of impingement or of rotator cuff rupture.

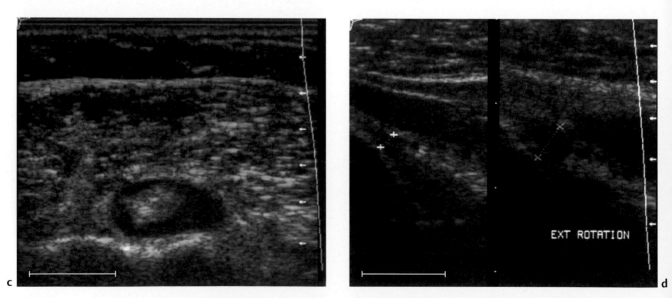

Fig. 173
A transverse scan at the level of the bicipital groove also shows fluid surrounding the biceps tendon (same patient as 173b). In external rotation, the posterior recess fills showing the joint effusion to a better extent (**c** and **d**).

Milwaukee Shoulder

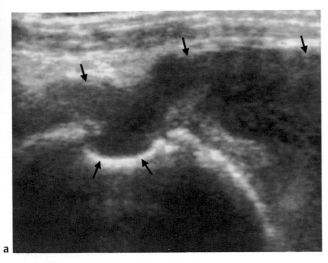

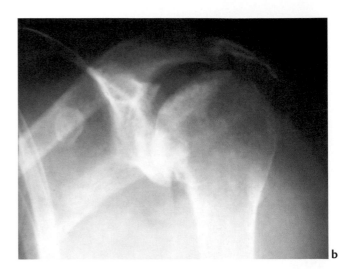

Fig. 174
Absent rotator cuff, hypoechoic effusion, and an erosion (→) at the external joint surface in a coronal plane (**a**). The corresponding plain film shows destruction of the glenohumeral joint and extensive subchondral sclerosis. Acromial changes and secondary osteochondromatosis are also seen (**b**).

Milwaukee shoulder syndrome is most commonly seen in elderly women. It corresponds to a destructive arthropathy, due to hydroxyapatite or mixed calcium phosphate crystal accumulation. Clinical signs are often mild in comparison with the plain film findings, which are cartilage and osseous destruction, subchondral sclerosis, intra-articular debris, rotator cuff rupture, joint disorganization or deformity. Some authors believe that the initial alteration is a disruption of rotator cuff, allowing ascension of the humeral head.

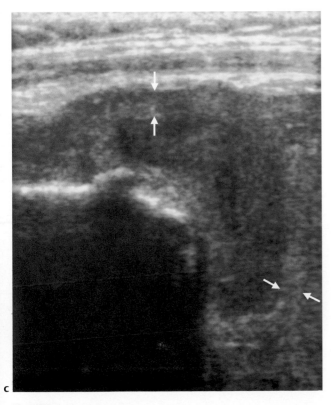

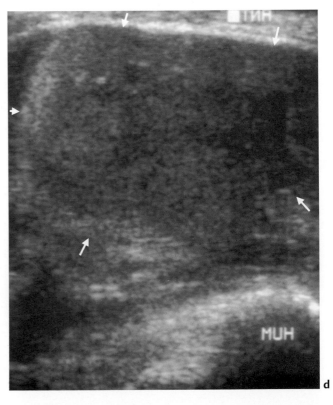

Fig. 174
A thickened wall of the bursa (→) and its hypoechoic content are shown on this coronal view at the level of the greater tuberosity (**c**). An anterior axial scan of the proximal humerus shows a distended subdeltoid bursa (→) with echoic contents. Blood was aspirated from this bursa (**d**).

Shoulder

Traumatic Injury

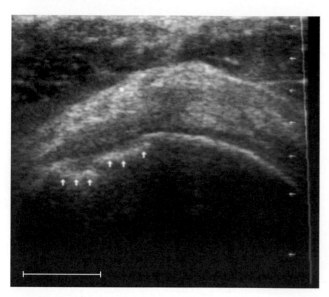

Fig. 175
An axial scan shows a depressed articular surface at the posterior part of the humeral head, corresponding to a small Hill–Sachs lesion (→).

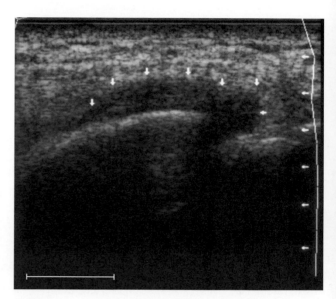

Fig. 176
A tender and distended hypoechoic capsule (→) of the acromioclavicular joint corresponds to a grade I acromioclavicular luxation in this patient, following a bicycle injury.

Ultrasound is useful in the evaluation of complications after shoulder dislocation. Anterior dislocations represent 95% of dislocations. They can be complicated by greater tuberosity fractures and rotator cuff tear or avulsion (20–50 % of cases) or by Hill–Sachs deformity (21% of dislocations and 74% of recurrent dislocations), appearing as a wedge- shaped defect of the posterolateral aspect of the humeral head, corresponding to a compression fracture of this zone against the glenoid rim. Another complication is myositis ossifi-

cans. Posterior dislocations are rare, but can be associated with compression fracture of the humeral head or of the lesser tuberosity. Acromioclavicular sprain is also a frequent traumatic pathology of the shoulder. Grade II (elevation of the clavicle by less than its width) and grade III (elevation of the clavicle above the superior aspect of the acromion) are easily diagnosed on a plain film. Grade I, with only soft tissue swelling, is more easily confirmed by ultrasound.

Anatomy

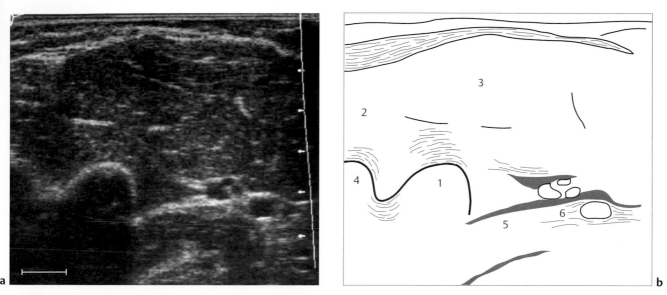

Fig. 177
Anterior transverse scan of the middle third. Humerus (**1**), brachialis (**2**), biceps (**3**), triceps lateral head (**4**), triceps medial head (**5**) muscle, brachial vessels (**6**) (**a** and **b**).

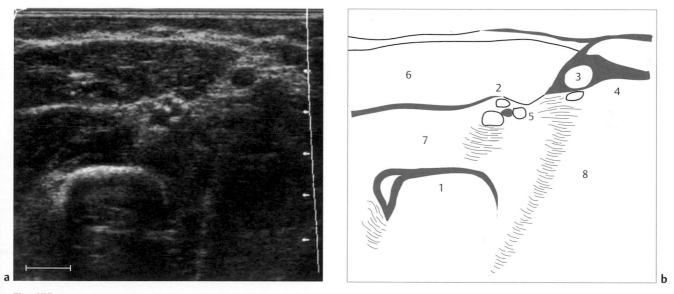

Fig. 178
Antero-medial transverse scan of the distal third. Humerus (**1**), brachial artery (**2**), basilar vein (**3**), cubital nerve (**4**), brachial nerve (**5**), biceps (**6**), brachialis (**7**), medial head of triceps (**8**) muscle (**a** and **b**).

Upper Arm

Anatomy

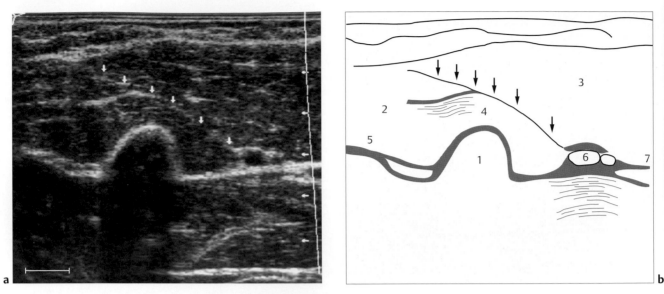

Fig. 179
Posterior transverse scan of the middle third. Humerus (**1**), triceps muscle : lateral head (**2**), long head (**3**), medial head (**4**), lateral intermuscular septum (**5**), brachial artery (**6**), medial intermuscular septum (**7**) (**a** and **b**).

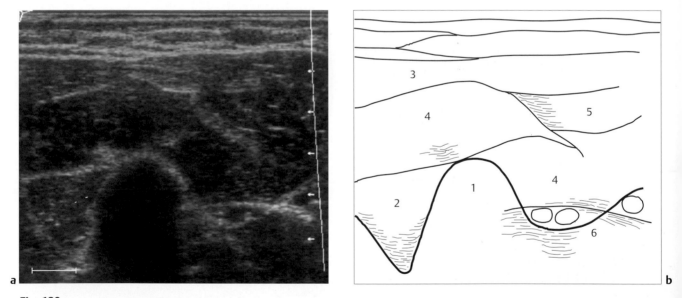

Fig. 180
Posterior transverse scan of the distal third. Humerus (**1**), brachialis (**2**), triceps muscle : lateral head (**3**), medial head (**4**), long head (**5**), vessel and nerve (**6**) (**a** and **b**).

Anatomy

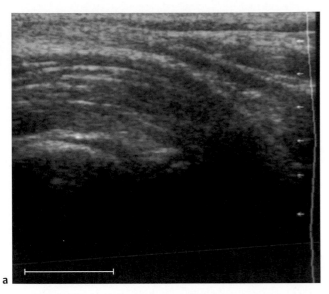 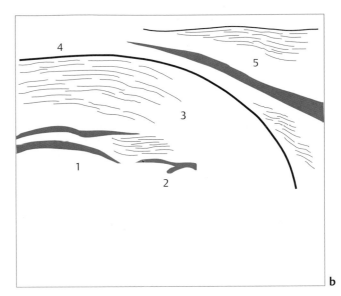

Fig. 181
Medial sagittal scan. Trochlea (**1**), coronoid process (**2**), brachialis (**3**), biceps (**4**), brachioradialis (**5**) muscle (**a** and **b**).

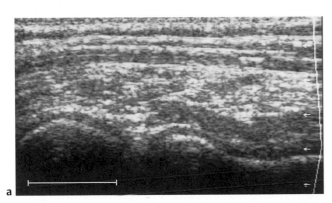 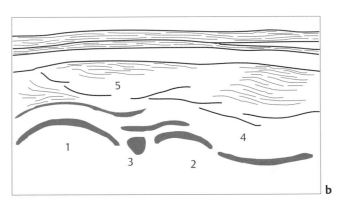

Fig. 182
Anterior sagittal scan at the level of the radiohumeral joint. Capitulum (**1**), radius (**2**), annular ligament (**3**), supinator (**4**), brachioradialis (**5**) muscle (**a** and **b**).

The anterior fat pad overlies the coronoid fossa and is pressed into it by the brachialis tendon during extension of the elbow. When examining the posterior fat pad, the elbow should be flexed to avoid spurious elevation of the fat pad.

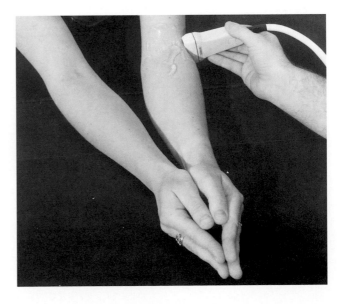

Fig. 183
Position for the evaluation of the insertion of the extensor tendons.

Elbow

Anatomy

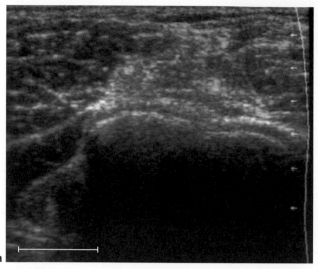 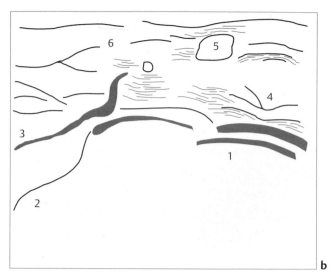

Fig. 184
Anterolateral transverse scan. Capitulum (**1**), extensor digitorum (**2**), extensor carpi radialis longus (**3**), brachialis (**4**), biceps (**5**), brachioradialis muscle (**6**) (**a** and **b**).

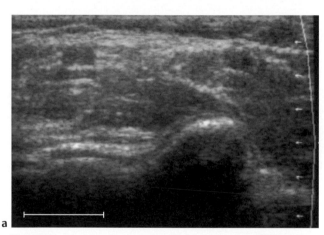 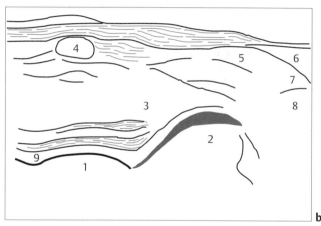

Fig. 185
Anteromedial transverse scan. Capitulum (**1**), trochlea (**2**), brachialis muscle (**3**), brachial artery (**4**), pronator teres (**5**), flexor carpi radialis (**6**), palmaris longus (**7**), flexor digitorum superficialis (**8**) muscle, cartilage (**9**) (**a** and **b**).

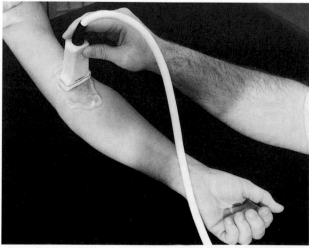

Fig. 186
Position for the anterior evaluation of the elbow.

On transverse views, the brachioradialis, biceps, brachialis, and pronator teres muscles are visible as hypoechoic cross sections anterior to the humerus at its radial, medial, and ulnar aspects, respectively. On sagittal views, these muscles are seen to arch over the joint. The elbow should be examined anteriorly in a comparative way on full extension and supination. Anterior articular recesses, bone surfaces, muscles, and tendons can be seen in this position. The median nerve is located between the pronator teres and the brachialis muscles. The radial nerve is found between the biceps tendon and the extensor muscles. The lateral epicondyle is evaluated in a semipronated position.

Anatomy

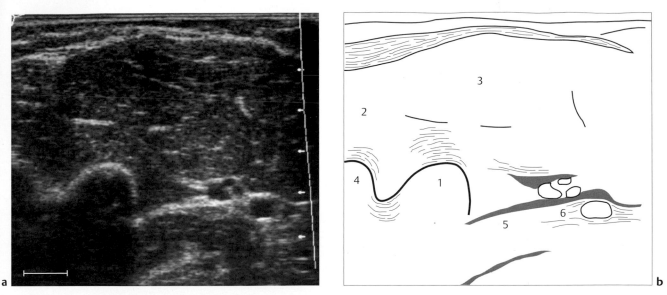

Fig. 177
Anterior transverse scan of the middle third. Humerus (**1**), brachialis (**2**), biceps (**3**), triceps lateral head (**4**), triceps medial head (**5**) muscle, brachial vessels (**6**) (**a** and **b**).

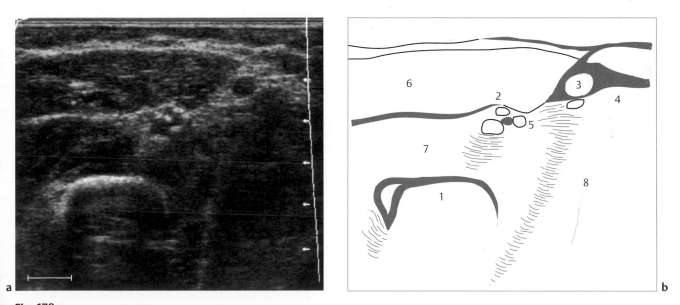

Fig. 178
Antero-medial transverse scan of the distal third. Humerus (**1**), brachial artery (**2**), basilar vein (**3**), cubital nerve (**4**), brachial nerve (**5**), biceps (**6**), brachialis (**7**), medial head of triceps (**8**) muscle (**a** and **b**).

Upper Arm

Anatomy

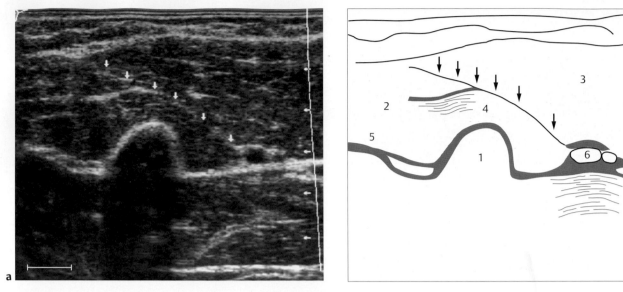

Fig. 179
Posterior transverse scan of the middle third. Humerus (**1**), triceps muscle : lateral head (**2**), long head (**3**), medial head (**4**), lateral intermuscular septum (**5**), brachial artery (**6**), medial intermuscular septum (**7**) (**a** and **b**).

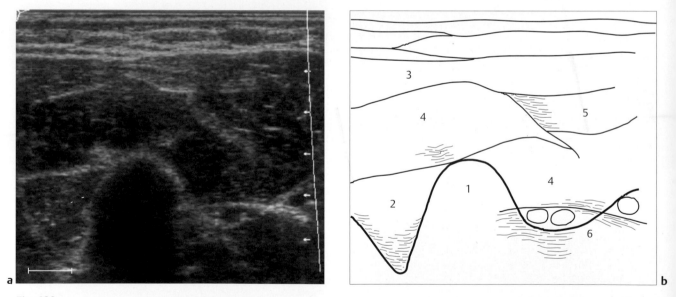

Fig. 180
Posterior transverse scan of the distal third. Humerus (**1**), brachialis (**2**), triceps muscle : lateral head (**3**), medial head (**4**), long head (**5**), vessel and nerve (**6**) (**a** and **b**).

Anatomy

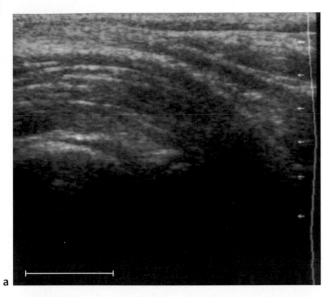
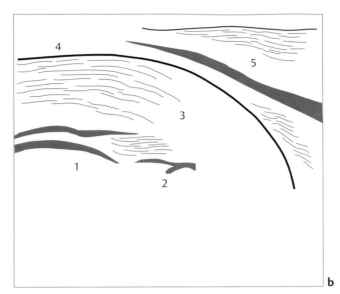

Fig. 181
Medial sagittal scan. Trochlea (**1**), coronoid process (**2**), brachialis (**3**), biceps (**4**), brachioradialis (**5**) muscle (**a** and **b**).

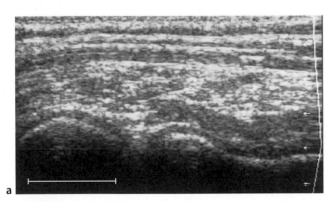
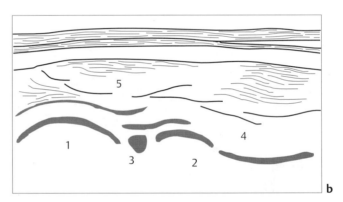

Fig. 182
Anterior sagittal scan at the level of the radiohumeral joint. Capitulum (**1**), radius (**2**), annular ligament (**3**), supinator (**4**), brachioradialis (**5**) muscle (**a** and **b**).

The anterior fat pad overlies the coronoid fossa and is pressed into it by the brachialis tendon during extension of the elbow. When examining the posterior fat pad, the elbow should be flexed to avoid spurious elevation of the fat pad.

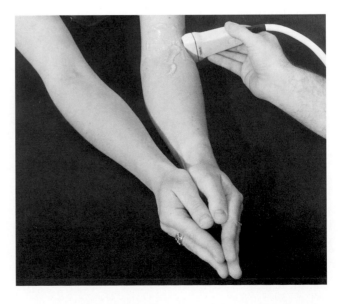

Fig. 183
Position for the evaluation of the insertion of the extensor tendons.

Elbow

Anatomy

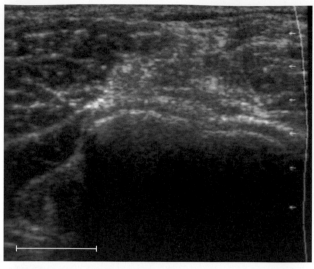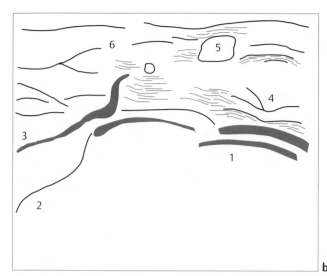

Fig. 184
Anterolateral transverse scan. Capitulum (**1**), extensor digitorum (**2**), extensor carpi radialis longus (**3**), brachialis (**4**), biceps (**5**), brachioradialis muscle (**6**) (**a** and **b**).

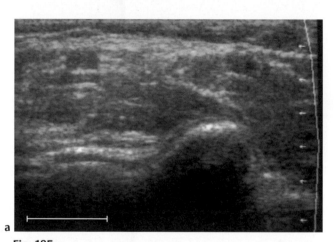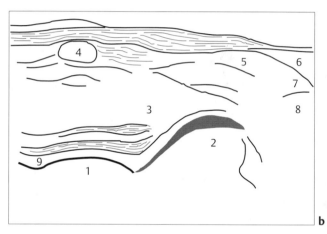

Fig. 185
Anteromedial transverse scan. Capitulum (**1**), trochlea (**2**), brachialis muscle (**3**), brachial artery (**4**), pronator teres (**5**), flexor carpi radialis (**6**), palmaris longus (**7**), flexor digitorum superficialis (**8**) muscle, cartilage (**9**) (**a** and **b**).

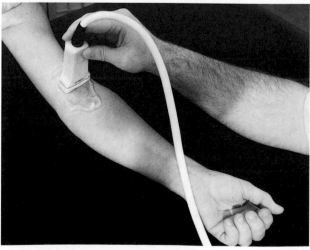

Fig. 186
Position for the anterior evaluation of the elbow.

On transverse views, the brachioradialis, biceps, brachialis, and pronator teres muscles are visible as hypoechoic cross sections anterior to the humerus at its radial, medial, and ulnar aspects, respectively. On sagittal views, these muscles are seen to arch over the joint. The elbow should be examined anteriorly in a comparative way on full extension and supination. Anterior articular recesses, bone surfaces, muscles, and tendons can be seen in this position. The median nerve is located between the pronator teres and the brachialis muscles. The radial nerve is found between the biceps tendon and the extensor muscles. The lateral epicondyle is evaluated in a semipronated position.

Anatomy

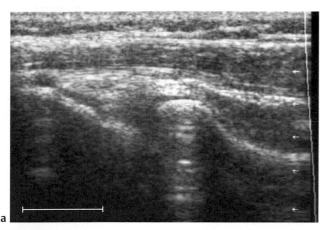
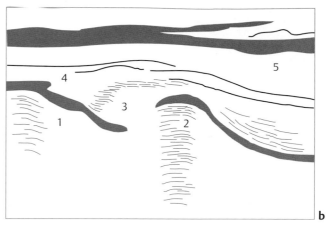

Fig. 187
Sagittal scan of the lateral epicondyle and the radial head. Lateral epicondyle (**1**), radial head (**2**), annular lateral collateral ligament (**3**), extensor digitorum tendon (**4**), extensor carpi radialis longus muscle (**5**) (**a** and **b**).

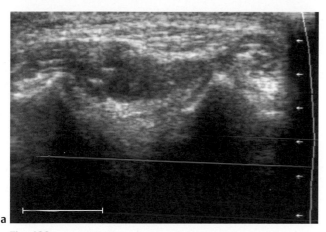
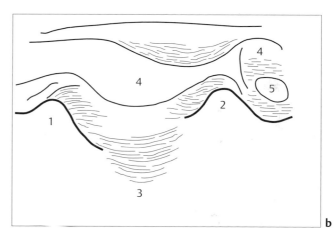

Fig. 188
Posteromedial transverse scan. Lateral epicondyle (**1**), medial epicondyle (**2**), olecranon fossa (**3**), triceps muscle (**4**), ulnar nerve (**5**) (**a** and **b**).

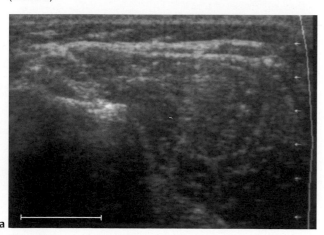
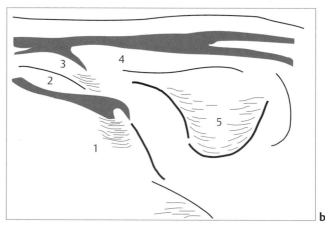

Fig. 189
Posterior transverse scan of the capitulum (**1**), common extensor tendon (2), extensor digitorum (3), extensor carpi radialis longus and brevis (**4**), brachioradialis (**5**) muscle (**a** and **b**).

The common flexor tendon at the medial epicondyle and the common extensor tendon at the lateral epicondyle are covered by the hyperechoic medial and lateral collateral ligaments, which form the articular capsule. The lateral collateral ligament is inseparable from the annular ligament; they appear hyperechoic and invaginate between the radial head and the lateral epicondyle.

Elbow

Anatomy

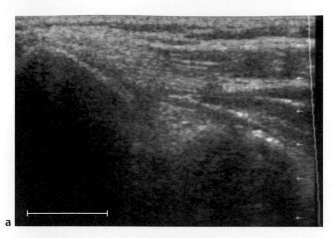
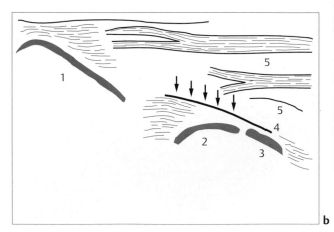

a   b

Fig. 190
Coronal scan of the medial epicondyle. Medial epicondyle (**1**), trochlea (**2**), coronoid process (**3**), medial radial collateral ligament (→) (**4**), flexor digitorum muscle (**5**) (**a** and **b**).

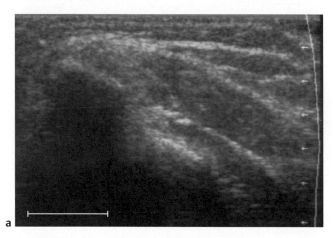
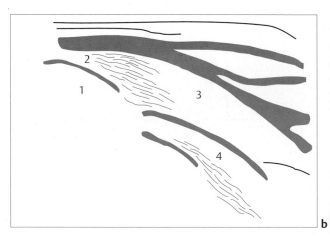

a   b

Fig. 191
Medial coronal scan. Trochlea (**1**), common flexor tendon (**2**), pronator teres (**3**), brachialis muscle (**4**) (**a** and **b**).

Anterior and posterior fat pads appear as echoic triangular structures lying within the coronoid and olecranon fossae. The posterior fat pad is larger or of the same size as the anterior one. The articular cartilage over the capitulum and the trochlea is seen as a thin hypoechoic line between the fat pad and the bone. The fat pads around the elbow joint lie between the fibrous capsule and the synovial membrane. The posterior fat pad is the largest, overlying the olecranon fossa, into which it is pressed by the triceps tendon upon flexion of the elbow.

Anatomy

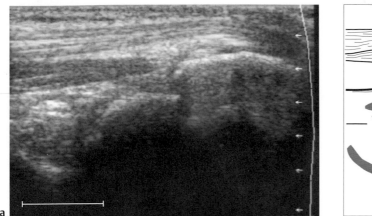
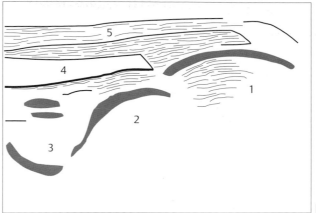

Fig. 192
Posterior longitudinal scan of the olecranon. Olecranon (**1**), trochlea (**2**), olecranon fossa (**3**), triceps muscle (**4**), triceps tendon (**5**) (**a** and **b**).

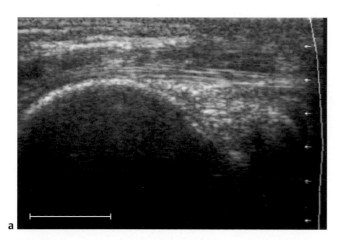
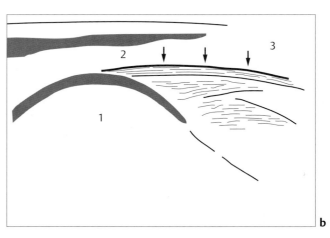

Fig. 193
Posteromedial longitudinal scan. Medial epicondyle (1), ulnar nerve (→) (2), triceps muscle (3) (**a** and **b**).

From posterior, the ulnar nerve is seen as a hyperechoic fibrillar structure, medial to the olecranon fossa and lying on the posterior border of the medial epicondyle. More distally, the nerve is situated in the middle of the triangle formed by the flexor digitorum superficialis muscle anteriorly, the flexor digitorum profundus muscle posteriorly, and the flexor carpi ulnaris muscle medially. The hyperechoic triceps tendon insertion into the olecranon is easily identified in a posterior sagittal view.

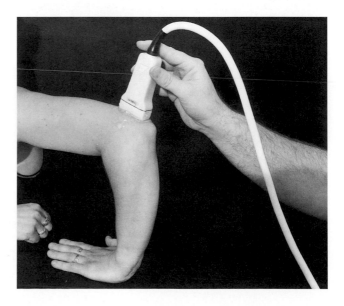

Fig. 194
Position for the posterior evaluation of the elbow.

Elbow

Effusion and Loose Bodies

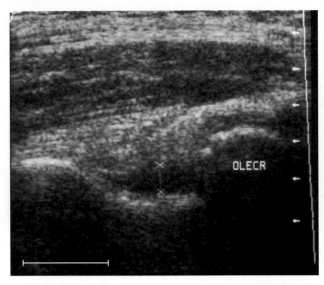

Fig. 195
A small amount of anechoic fluid is shown in the olecranon fossa (posterior approach).

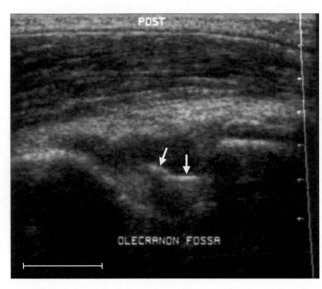

Fig. 196
Loose bodies (→) are found in a fluid-filled olecranon fossa.

Effusion of the elbow can be recognized by examination of the anterior synovial recess, which is demonstrated on a longitudinal scan of the anterior aspect of the elbow in complete extension. Under normal conditions, there is only a fluid film between the capsule and the articular cartilage. If the fluid is more than 1 mm thick, larger effusion is present. In this case, examination of the joint recess is mandatory to detect intra-articular loose bodies.

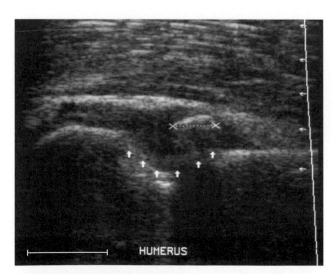

Fig. 197
Fluid and a loose body are seen in the coronoid fossa (→) (anterior approach) in this sagittal plane at the level of the distal humerus.

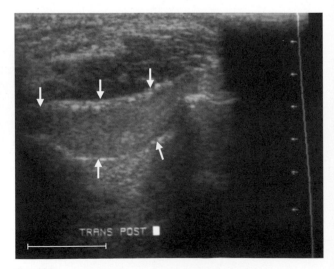

Fig. 198
Acute hyperechoic hemarthrosis (→) seen in the olecranon fossa on a transverse scan.

Olecranon Bursitis

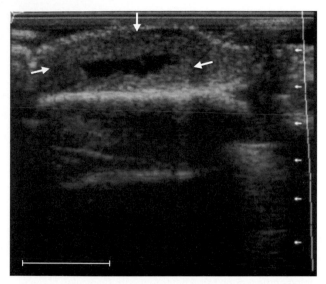

Fig. 199
Sagittal scan shows a chronic frictional bursitis (→), with anechoic contents and a thickened echoic wall.

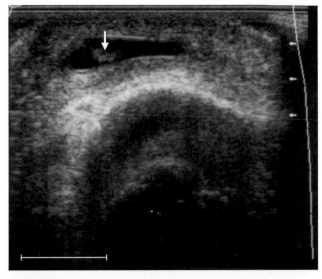

Fig. 200
A transverse scan shows a bursitis with a wall indistinguishable from the surrounding fat due to diffuse inflammatory changes. A tophaceous nodule (→) is found in the anechoic content of the bursitis in this patient with gout.

Olecranon bursitis is a frequent condition. It appears as a fluid collection limited by the synovial wall, and of variable thickness and appearance. The content can be hypoechoic or anechoic as in frictional bursitis, or hyperechoic as in infectious or metabolic bursitis. In chronic gout, the bursa often contains hyperechoic nodules that can calcify.

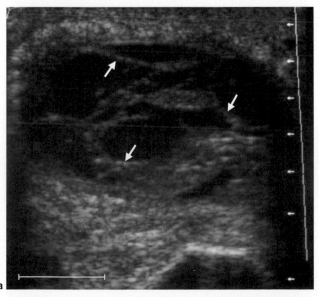

a b

Fig. 201
This chronic gouty bursitis is septated (→) on a transverse scan (**a**), and contains hyperechoic nodules (**b**).

Elbow

Lateral Epicondylitis

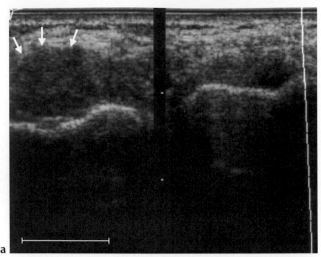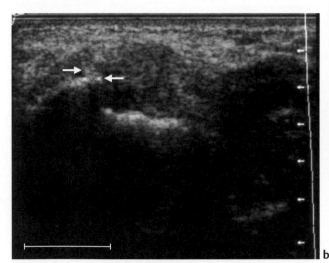

a
b

Fig. 202
A comparative study of the lateral epicondyles shows unilateral thickening of the tendon (**a**). A heterogeneous thickening of the tendon was found, with a hyperechoic focus causing an acoustic shadow (→), compatible with a calcification (**b**).

Lateral epicondylitis is also called "tennis elbow", and corresponds to a tendinitis of the extensor muscles that insert on the lateral epicondyle. It is the most frequent tendinitis of the elbow. In normal individuals, the tendon appears as a hyperechoic triangle. Bilateral examination will show the hypoechoic appearance and the thickening of the tendon compared to the contralateral side. The tendon can be heterogeneous and contain calcifications, and intrasubstance ruptures can be seen as anechoic lines. The examination should include the proximal part of the muscle, which can show focal alterations.

Medial Epicondylitis

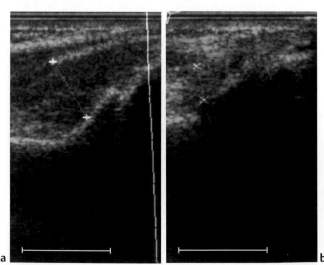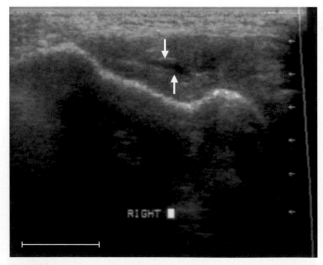

a
b

Fig. 203
Thickening and hypoechoic appearance (→) of the flexor muscles at their insertion. The contralateral insertion is normal (**a** and **b**).

Fig. 204
A small linear anechoic rupture (→) in medial epicondylitis.

Medial epicondylitis, "golfer's elbow", corresponds to a tendinitis of the ulnar flexor muscles. It is less frequent than lateral epicondylitis. The ultrasound characteristics are the same as in other forms of tendinitis, with thickening of the tendon and a hypoechoic, heterogeneous appearance. The diagnosis is made by comparison with the contralateral side.

Biceps and Triceps Tendon Pathology

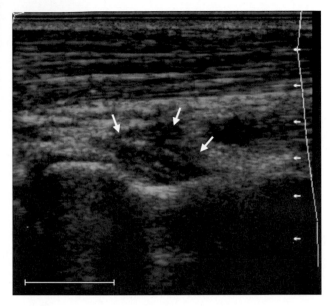

Fig. 205
A thickened hypoechoic distal biceps tendon (→) close to the insertion on the bicipital tuberosity, covered by the pronator teres muscle.

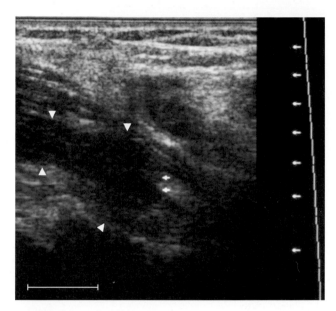

Fig. 206
Rupture of the biceps tendon is seen as a hypoechoic interruption (▶) deep to the brachioradialis muscle. The hyperechoic distal end is retracted (→).

In tendinitis, the biceps and triceps tendons can be swollen, heterogeneous, or hypoechoic. When they are ruptured, anechoic or hypoechoic clefts will be seen, with or without retraction of the free ends. A calcified enthesophyte is frequently found at the insertion of the triceps tendon on the olecranon, and is of traumatic or degenerative origin, or caused by a preexisting hyperostotic diathesis.

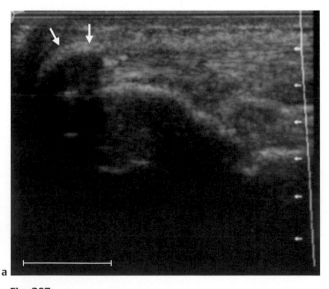

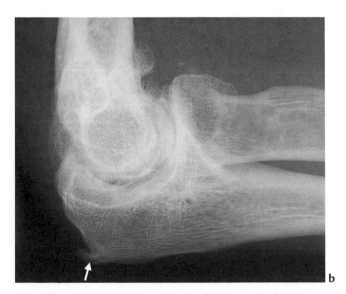

Fig. 207
The hyperechoic calcified insertion of the triceps tendon (→) on the olecranon (**a**) corresponds to an enthesophyte (→) on the plain film (**b**).

Ulnar Nerve Entrapment

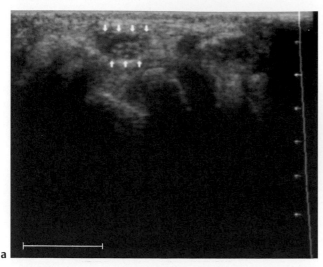

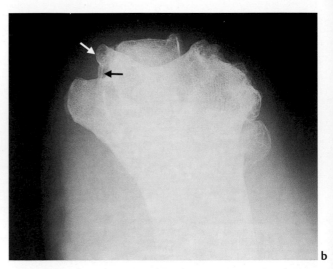

a

b

Fig. 208
The ulnar nerve showing a hypoechoic contour (→) is displaced, due to bone irregularities at the medial epicondyle (**a**) also seen on the plain film (→) (**b**).

The ulnar nerve can easily be identified in its groove at the posterior aspect of the medial epicondyle. Bony excrescences of posttraumatic or degenerative origin, or tumoral processes such as cysts or synovial prolif-eration in patients with rheumatoid arthritis can induce ulnar nerve irritation due to entrapment or nerve displacement.

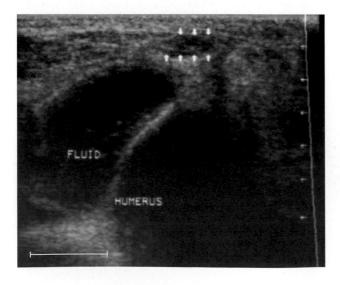

Fig. 209
An arthrosynovial cyst formed at the posteromedial aspect of the elbow is responsible for displacement of the ulnar nerve (→).

Rheumatoid Arthritis

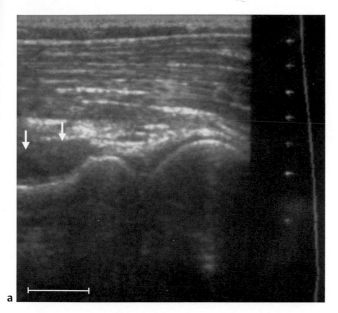

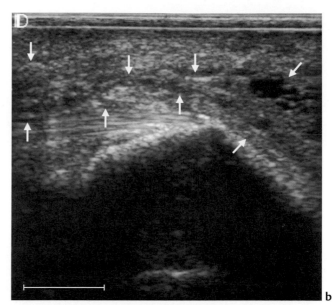

a
b

Fig. 210
A hypoechoic synovial proliferation is noted at the radial neck in this longitudinal scan (→) (**a**). A sagittal scan at the level of the olecranon shows a mixed echoic and anechoic bursitis (→) (**b**).

The elbow is frequently involved in rheumatoid arthritis. On ultrasound, effusion and synovial proliferation are seen. Pannus appears as a hypoechoic nodule. A bursitis can be associated, and show heterogeneous echoic contents. These signs can appear before osseous changes, and if bilateral, are suggestive of rheumatoid arthritis.

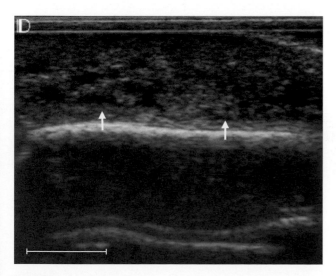

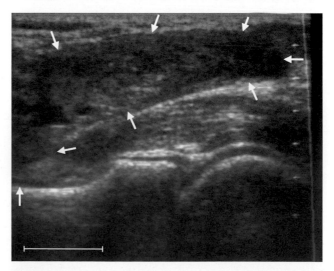

Fig. 211
A tranverse scan at the level of the olecranon shows a mixed echoic and anechoic bursitis (→).

Fig. 212
A heterogeneous mass located anterior to the radial neck corresponds to a rheumatoid nodule, arising from the annular recess (→).

Forearm

Anatomy

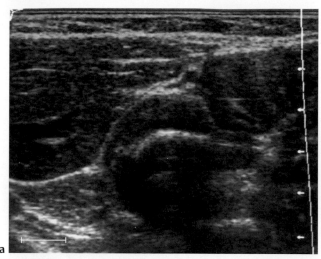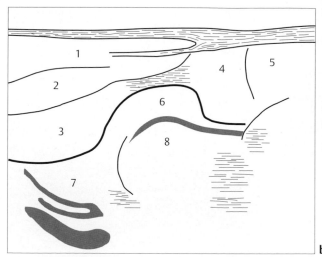

Fig. 213
Anterolateral transverse scan of the proximal third. Supinator (**1**), extensor carpi radialis longus (**2**), extensor carpi radialis brevis (**3**), pronator teres (**4**), palmaris longus (**5**), supinator deep portion (**6**), extensor digitorum (**7**) muscles, radius (**8**) (**a** and **b**).

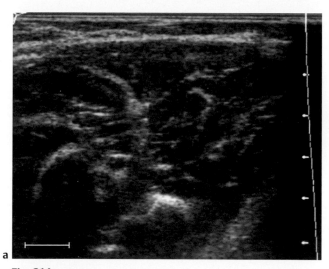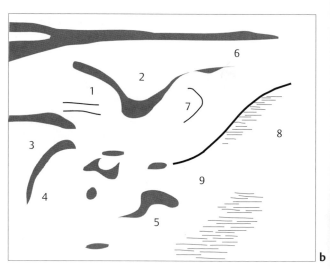

Fig. 214
Anteromedial transverse scan of the proximal third. Pronator teres (**1**), palmaris longus (**2**), supinator deep portion muscles (**3**), radius (**4**), ulna (**5**), palmaris brevis (**6**), flexor digitorum superficialis (**7**), flexor carpi ulnaris (**8**), flexor digitorum profundus (**9**) muscles (**a** and **b**).

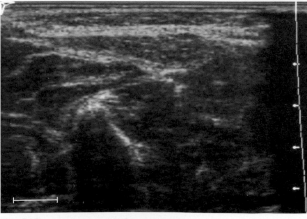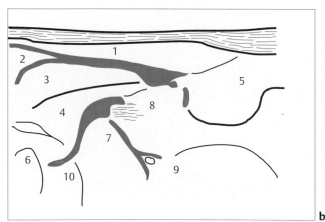

Fig. 215
Anterolateral transverse scan of the middle third. Supinator (**1**), extensor carpi radialis longus (**2**), extensor carpi radialis brevis (**3**), pronator teres (**4**), palmaris longus (**5**), extensor digitorum muscles (**6**), radius (**7**), flexor digitorum superficialis (**8**), flexor pollicis longus (**9**), abductor pollicis longus (**10**) muscles (**a** and **b**).

Anatomy

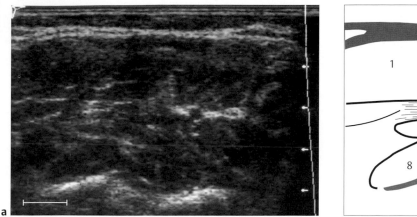
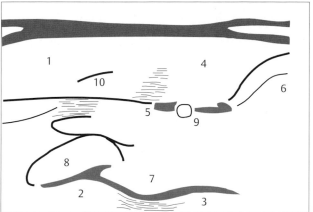

Fig. 216
Anteromedial transverse scan of the middle third. Palmaris longus muscle (**1**), radius (**2**), ulna (**3**), palmaris brevis (**4**), flexor digitorum superficialis (**5**), flexor carpi ulnaris (**6**), flexor digitorum profundus (**7**), flexor pollicis longus (**8**) muscles, ulnar artery (**9**), median nerve (**10**) (**a** and **b**).

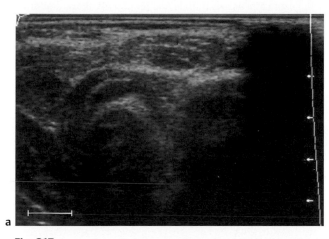
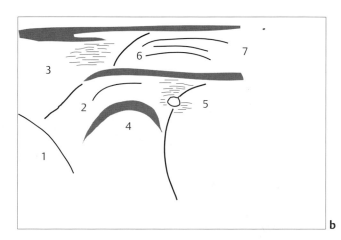

Fig. 217
Posterior transverse scan of the proximal third. Extensor carpi radialis brevis (**1**), supinator (**2**), extensor digitorum muscle (**3**), radius (**4**), ulna (**5**), extensor digiti minimi (**6**), extensor carpi ulnaris (**7**) muscles (**a** and **b**).

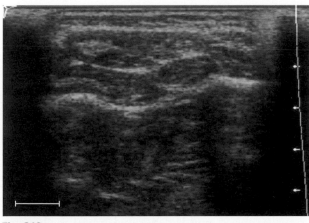
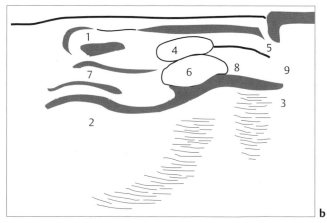

Fig. 218
Posterior transverse scan of the middle third. Extensor digitorum muscle (**1**), radius (**2**), ulna (**3**), extensor digiti minimi (**4**), extensor carpi ulnaris (**5**), extensor pollicis brevis (**6**), abductor pollicis longus (**7**), extensor pollicis longus (**8**), extensor indicis (**9**) muscles (**a** and **b**).

Wrist

Anatomy

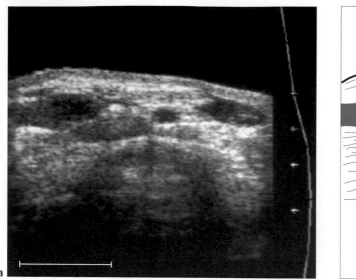
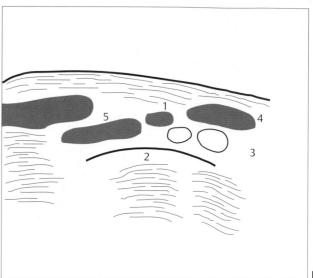

Fig. 219
Anteromedial transverse scan. Ulnar artery (**1**), ulna (**2**), ulnar nerve (**3**), flexor carpi ulnaris muscle and tendon (**4**), flexor digitorum tendons (**5**) (**a** and **b**).

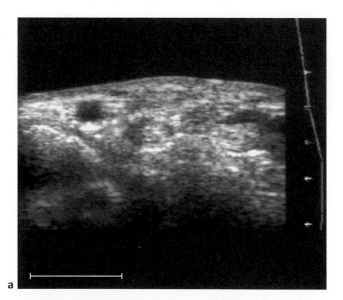
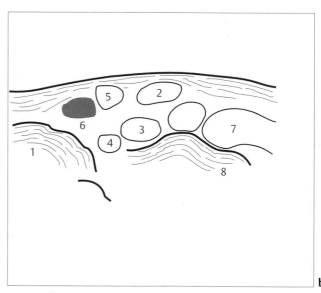

Fig. 220
Anterolateral transverse scan. Radius (**1**), palmaris longus tendon (**2**), median nerve (**3**), flexor pollicis longus tendon (**4**), flexor carpi radialis tendon (**5**), radial artery (**6**), flexor digitorum superficialis tendon (**7**), flexor digitorum profundus tendons (**8**) (**a** and **b**).

On the anterior aspect, the most medial tendon is the flexor carpi ulnaris, which runs superficial to the ulnar nerve. The ulnar artery is easily identified between these two structures and the most medial flexor tendons. The carpal tunnel is bordered anteriorly by the flexor retinaculum and contains three superficial and three deep flexor tendons, the flexor pollicis lon-gus tendon, and the median nerve in an anterolateral position. The palmaris longus tendon has a subcutaneous location in front of the median nerve. The flexor carpi radialis tendon has the most lateral position on a transverse scan and is separated from the abductor pollicis longus and extensor pollicis brevis tendon by the radial artery.

Anatomy

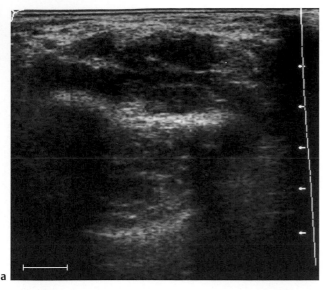 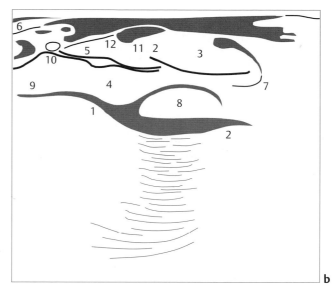

Fig. 221
Anterior transverse scan above the musculotendinous junction. Radius (**1**), ulna (**2**), flexor digitorum superficialis (**3**), flexor pollicis longus (**4**) muscles, median nerve (**5**), brachioradialis (**6**), flexor carpi ulnaris (**7**), flexor digitorum profundus (**8**), flexor pollicis longus (**9**) muscles, radial artery (**10**), flexor carpi radialis (**11**), palmaris longus (**12**) tendons (**a** and **b**).

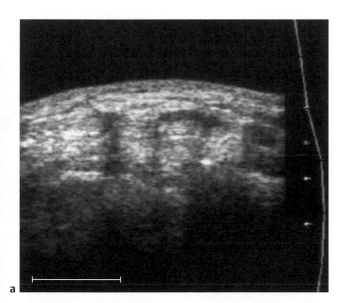 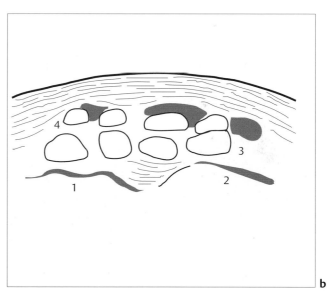

Fig. 222
Anterior transverse scan. Radius (**1**), ulna (**2**), flexor digitorum profundus (**3**), flexor digitorum superficialis and profundus tendons (**4**) (**a** and **b**).

The median nerve has a fibrillar texture, but is slightly less echoic than the flexor tendons. It is identified by its immobility, in contrast to the mobile adjacent tendons. The pronator quadratus muscle covers the radius and ulna anteriorly on more proximal transverse scans. At this level, the musculotendinous junctions are easily discerned from the hyperechoic nerves.

Anatomy

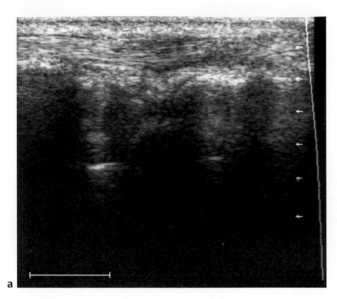
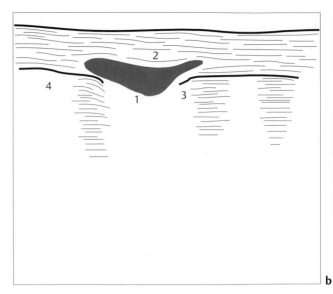

Fig. 223
Coronal scan of the medial aspect of the wrist. Triangular fibrocartilage and complex (**1**), extensor carpi ulnaris tendon (**2**), triquetrum (**3**), ulna (**4**) (**a** and **b**).

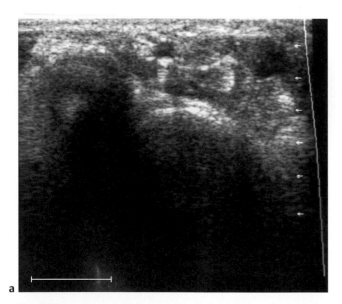
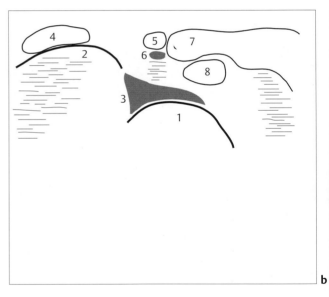

Fig. 224
Transverse scan of the anteromedial aspect at the level of the triangular fibrocartilage and complex. Radius (**1**), ulna (**2**), triangular fibrocartilage and complex (**3**), extensor carpi ulnaris tendon (**4**), ulnar artery (**5**), ulnar nerve (**6**), flexor carpi ulnaris muscle and tendon (**7**), flexor digitorum profundus tendon (**8**) (**a** and **b**).

On the lateral aspect of the radius, the extensor pollicis brevis and abductor pollicis longus tendons are identified. On the medial aspect, the hyperechoic triangular fibrocartilage complex can be evaluated in a coronal plane using the extensor carpi ulnaris tendon as a window. These structures can also be evaluated in a transverse plane. On the dorsal aspect of the distal radius, the radial tubercle can be used as a bone landmark. The extensor pollicis longus tendon lies in a groove of this protuberance.

Anatomy

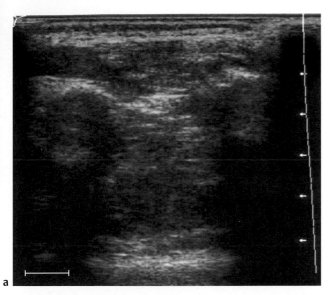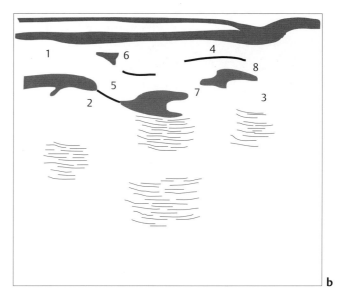

Fig. 225
Posterior transverse scan above the musculotendinous junction. Extensor digitorum muscle (**1**), radius (**2**), ulna (**3**), extensor carpi ulnaris (**4**), supinator (**5**), extensor digiti minimi (**6**), abductor pollicis longus (**7**), extensor pollicis longus (**8**) muscles (**a** and **b**).

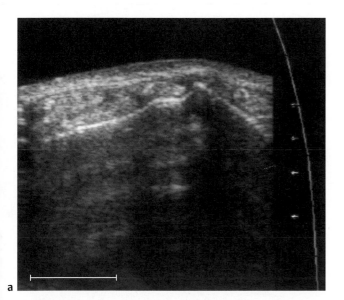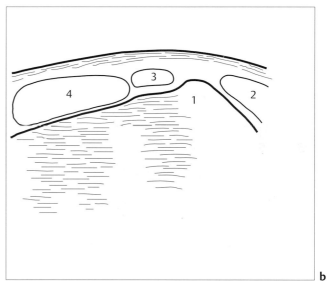

Fig. 226
Posterior transverse scan. Radius (**1**), extensor carpi radialis brevis and longus tendon (**2**), extensor pollicis longus tendon (**3**), extensor digitorum and indicis tendon (**4**) (**a** and **b**).

The extensor carpi radialis brevis and longus tendons can be identified lateral to the tubercle. The extensor digitorum and extensor indicis tendons, covered by the extensor retinaculum, are located medial to the tubercle. The extensor digiti minimi tendon has a more medial topography and runs on the posterior aspect of the radioulnar joint. The extensor carpi ulnaris tendon lies in a groove on the posteromedial aspect of the distal ulna and continues on the posterior aspect of the styloid process of the ulna and the triquetrum.

Anatomy

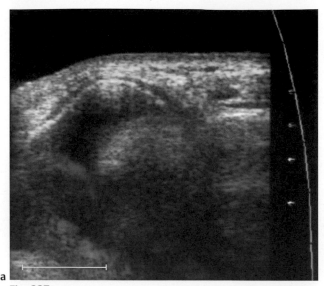
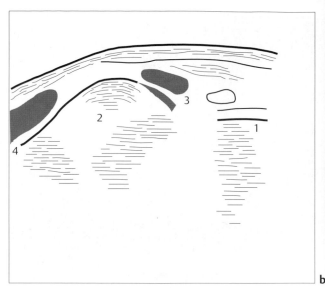

Fig. 227
Posteromedial transverse scan. Radius (**1**), ulna (**2**), extensor digiti minimi tendon (**3**), extensor carpi ulnaris tendon (**4**) (**a** and **b**).

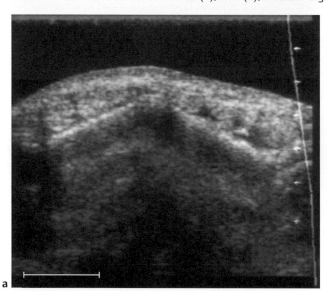
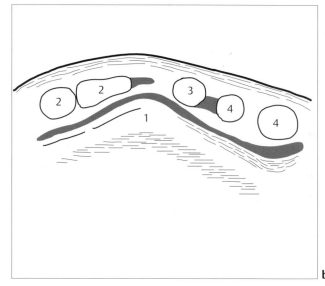

Fig. 228
Posterolateral transverse scan. Radius (**1**), extensor carpi radialis brevis and longus tendons (**2**), extensor pollicis longus tendon (**3**), extensor digitorum and indicis tendons (4) (**a** and **b**).

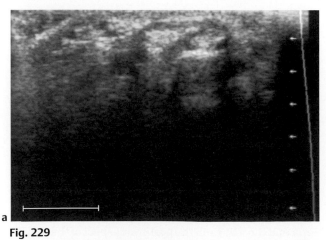
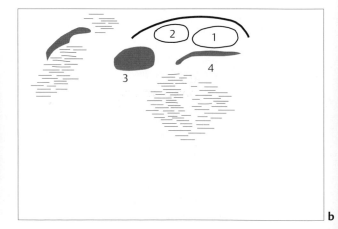

Fig. 229
Transverse scan of the lateral aspect of the wrist. Extensor pollicis brevis tendon (**1**), abductor pollicis longus tendon (**2**), radial artery (**3**), radius (**4**) (**a** and **b**).

Arthrosynovial Cyst

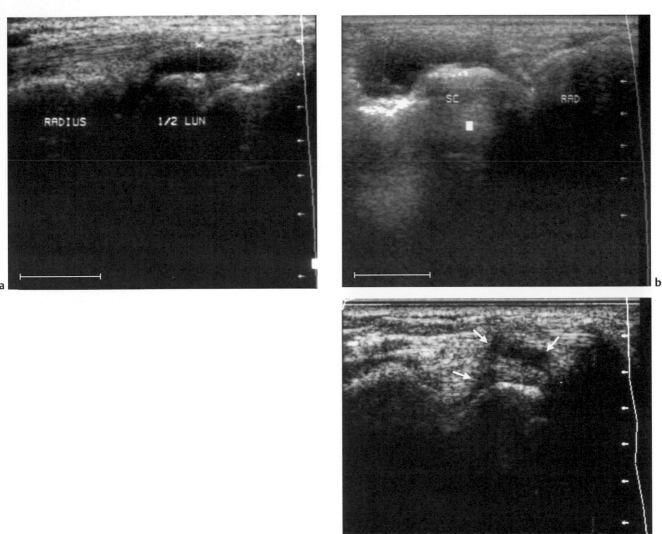

Fig. 230
Arthrosynovial cysts of various topographies are shown on a dorsal sagittal scan, with their articular communication making surgical planning easier: radiolunate cyst (**a**), radioscaphoid cyst (**b**), scaphotrapezoid cyst (**c**).

Arthrosynovial cysts are the most frequent cause of swelling of the wrist. They may develop from a joint or from a tendon sheath. Some of these cysts are so firm that their clinical diagnosis remains equivocal. They appear as anechoic or hypoechoic oval-shaped masses. Ultrasound shows the tendinous or articular communication, which is of interest in planning the surgical approach.

Wrist

Ganglion Cyst

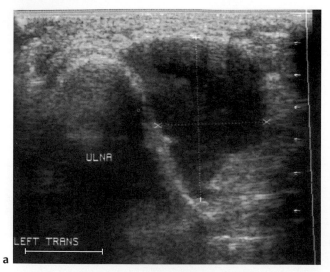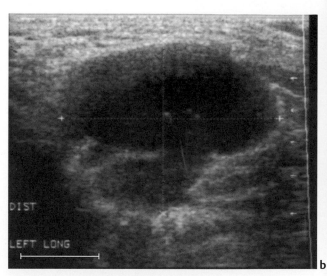

Fig. 231
A clinically obvious mass at the anteromedial border of the distal ulna presents on ultrasound as a thin-walled cystic lobulated lesion with internal echoes at the periphery. No significant posterior enhancement is noted (**a** and **b**).

Ganglion cysts are frequent in the wrist and appear as hypoechoic, or more often anechoic, round, oval, or lobulated masses. Their pathogenesis remains uncertain, and may include trauma, synovial herniation, or myxoid degeneration of connective tissue. Histologically, the wall of synovial cysts is made of compressed collagen fibers and flattened cells without a true synovial lining. Their content is viscous. They can communicate with the joint. Pain and tenderness are common symptoms. They may be associated with weakness or compressive neuropathy.

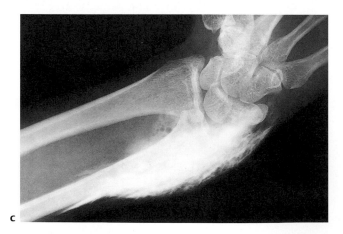

Fig. 231
Opacification of the lesion reveals no communication with joints or tendons (**c**).

Carpe Bossu

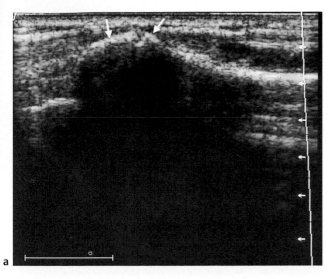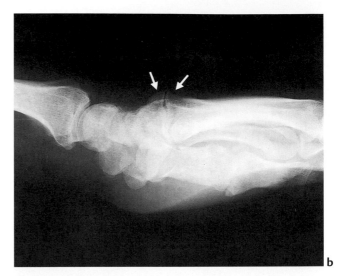

a

b

Fig. 232
A hypertrophied posterior cortex (→) at the base of the third metacarpal and adjacent distal capitate (**a**) correspond to a carpe bossu on plain film (→) (**b**).

In carpe bossu, the styloid process of the third meta-carpal and the adjacent capitate appear hypertrophic. Clinically, a firm swelling similar to a synovial cyst is felt. Ultrasound demonstrates the bony nature of the swelling, which shows as a hyperechoic band in continuity with the skeletal margins.

Scaphoid Fracture

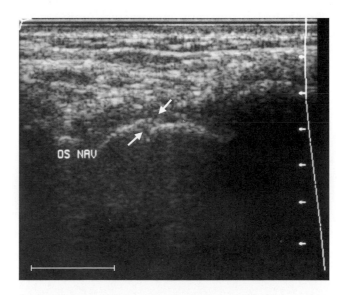

Fig. 233
A fracture of the middle third of the scaphoid is seen as an interrupted posterior cortex (→).

Ultrasound is capable of detecting small fractures, which appear as a discontinuity of the hyperechoic cortical line. This can be particularly useful in the early detection of scaphoid fractures, since they can be hard to find on plain films in the acute phase.

Gout

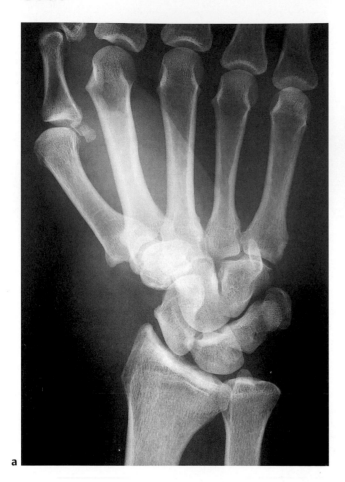

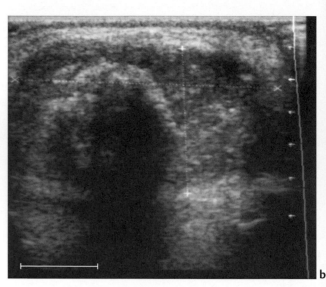

Fig. 234
This patient with chronic tophaceous gout presented with a tophus on the posterolateral aspect of the wrist seen on plain film (**a**). On ultrasound, the tophus was moderately echoic, containing central calcifications that caused an acoustic shadow (**b**).

In acute gouty arthritis, joint effusion is present, with moderate thickening of the synovial membrane. In chronic tophaceous gout, monosodium urate crystal deposition can occur in the periarticular soft tissue, in ligaments, bursae, and tendons, especially at the ex-

tensor side of the joint, where intense friction occurs. As they enlarge, tophi may calcify. Tophi appear as moderately echoic masses in the periarticular soft tissues.

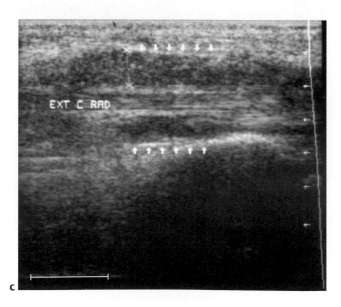

Fig. 234
Ultrasound shows oval-shaped echoic deposits (→) in the tendon sheath of the extensor carpi radialis muscle (**c**).

De Quervain's Tenosynovitis

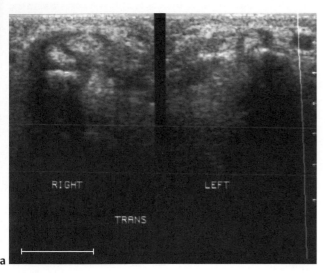
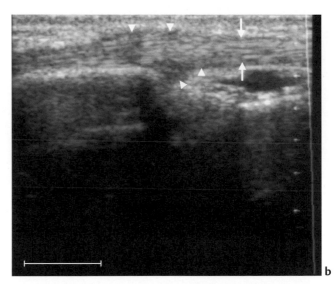

Fig. 235
Comparative image of a transverse scan at the outer border of the distal radius. De Quervain's tenosynovitis is present on the right, with tendon thickening and fluid accumulation in the synovial sheath (**a**). A longitudinal scan of the same patient shows tendon (→) and sheath (▶) thickening (**b**).

De Quervain's tenosynovitis is a chronic stenosing tenosynovitis of the tendons of the abductor pollicis longus and extensor pollicis brevis muscles. On transverse scans, a hypoechoic halo surrounds the tendons.

A comparison with the contralateral side is necessary to make the diagnosis, and the pathology is sometimes only found at the musculotendinous junction.

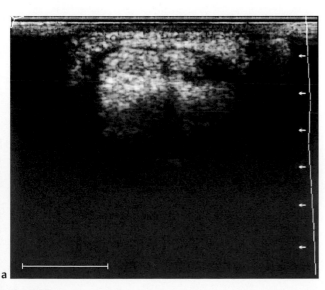
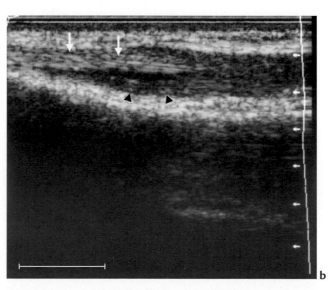

Fig. 236
A hypoechoic halo surrounds both tendons in a De Quervain's tenosynovitis (**a**). The musculotendinous junction has to be explored to make the diagnosis of the more proximal variant of De Quervain's tenosynovitis. Anechoic fluid is interposed between tendon (→) and muscle (▶) at this level (**b**).

Wrist

Tendinitis and Tenosynovitis

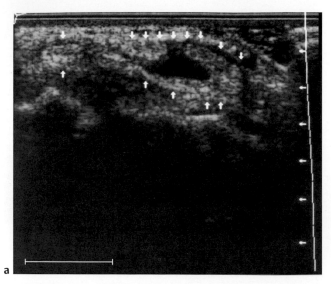
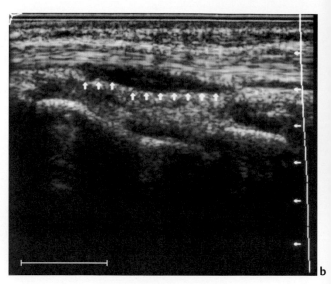

Fig. 237
This patient presented with tenosynovitis of the extensor digitorum and extensor indicis tendons, with a distended common tendon sheath and thickening of the tendons (→), shown on a transverse (**a**) and a longitudinal scan (→) (**b**).

At the level of the wrist, the tendons have synovial sheaths, which can contain several tendons. Tendon pain corresponds usually to tenosynovitis; tendinitis without tenosynovitis does not exist. In acute tenosynovitis, tendons can be swollen, and their sheaths are distended by anechoic fluid. In chronic, hemorrhagic, infectious, or rheumatoid tenosynovitis, fluid contains echoes. Tendons are better evaluated on a transverse scan.

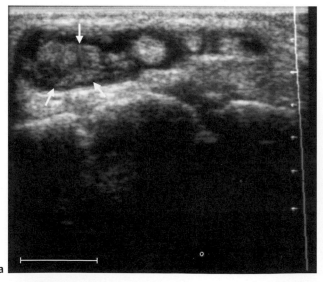
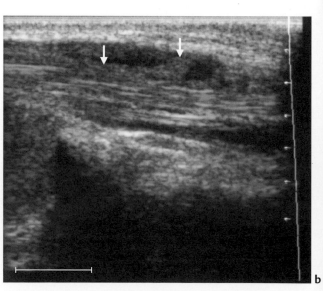

Fig. 238
A hemodialysis patient presented with hemorrhagic tenosynovitis of the extensor tendon. The effusion in the tendon sheath contains echoic foci (→) on transverse (**a**) and longitudinal (**b**) scans. A bloody effusion was aspirated. Traumatic hemorrhagic tenosynovitis has a similar appearance.

Rheumatoid Arthritis

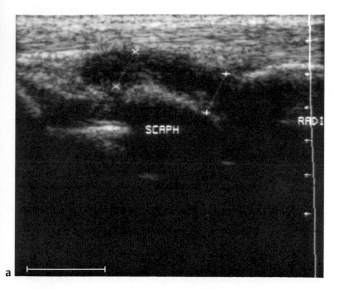
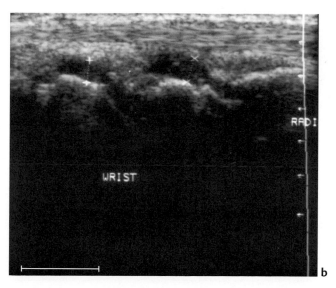

Fig. 239
Effusion with hypoechoic synovial proliferation is shown in a sagittal plane on the dorsum of the wrist at the level of the radioscaphoid (**a**), radiolunate and the lunocapitate joints (**b**).

Ultrasound may be useful in evaluating soft-tissue changes in the early stages of rheumatoid arthritis, when radiographic signs are subtle or absent. Ultrasound detects joint effusion. Synovial swelling around the ulnar styloid process appears as a hypoechoic mass, typically bilateral. Evaluation of the tendons is decisive, as their involvement can lead to rupture, giv-ing rise to the typical deformities of rheumatoid arthritis. Enlarged tendon sheaths are seen as oval or spindle-shaped cavities containing the hyperechoic tendon. The fluid contents are usually moderately echoic. Both longitudinal and transverse evaluations of the tendon structure are required. The rheumatoid nodules appear as small, rounded hypoechoic masses.

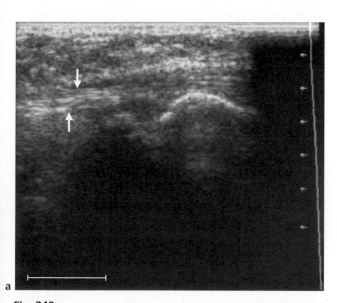
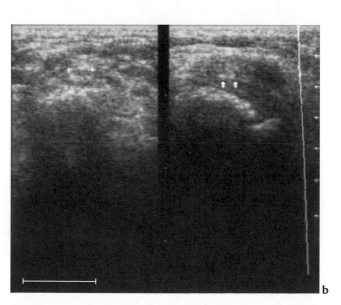

Fig. 240
Synovial proliferation of the tendon sheaths of the extensor carpi ulnaris tendon is seen as a hypoechoic ovoid mass surrounding and penetrating the tendon (→) in a longitudinal scan (**a**). Evaluation in a transverse plane shows the significant hypoechoic pannus. Only a few hyperechoic fibers remain intact at its center (→) (**b**).

Guyon's Canal Syndrome

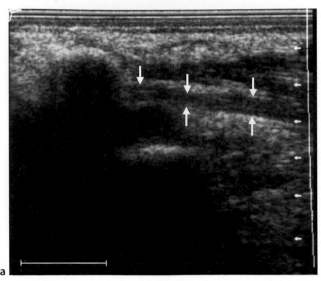
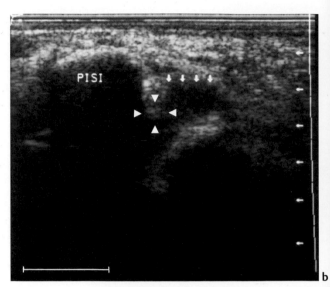

Fig. 241
A sagittal scan shows a cyst at the pisiform triquetrous joint compressing the ulnar nerve. The flexor carpi ulnaris tendon has a parallel course above the nerve (→) (**a**). The axial image of the same case shows the ulnar nerve (▶) compressed between the pisiform and the cyst (→) (**b**).

Entrapment of the ulnar nerve may occur in the canal of Guyon, where the nerve enters the wrist. The most frequent causes of this syndrome are ganglia and trauma.

Carpal Tunnel Syndrome

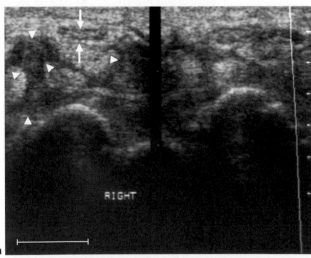
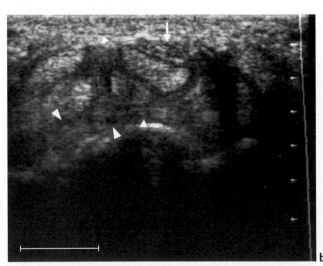

Fig. 242
Hypoechoic and flattened appearance of the median nerve (→) (**a**). The flexor retinaculum is bowed anteriorly, a hypoechoic tophus (▶) infiltrates the spaces around the flexor tendons in this patient with gout (**b**). The tendons are better revealed due to the tophus.

The median nerve is fibrillar in nature, but is less echoic than the surrounding tendons, and easily identified when the patient moves the digits. It is located just below the hyperechoic flexor retinaculum, along the axis of the second or the third finger. Characteristic ultrasound findings in carpal tunnel syndrome are: swelling of the median nerve in the proximal part of the carpal tunnel, nerve flattening in the distal part of the carpal tunnel, and increased bowing of the flexor retinaculum. These signs are not necessarily all present simultaneously.

Triangular Fibrocartilage Tear

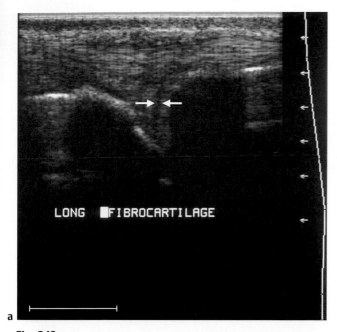
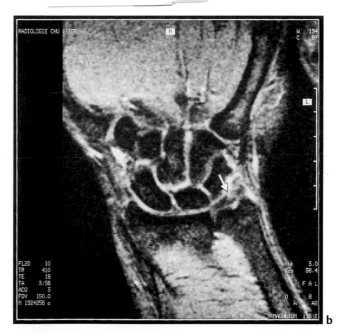

Fig. 243
A longitudinal medial scan showing a hypoechoic cleft (→) in the hyperechoic triangular fibrocartilage (**a**). The T_2-weighted MRI of the same patient in a frontal plane shows a hyperintense signal (→) in the triangular fibrocartilage (**b**).

The triangular fibrocartilage can be seen as a hyperechoic band located between the ulnar process, the radius, and the carpal bones. It can be scanned transversely by a palmar approach or longitudinally by a medial approach. In the latter, the extensor carpi ulnaris tendon can be used as a window. Fissures are seen as hypoechoic defects in the fibro-cartilage.

Wrist

Amyloidosis

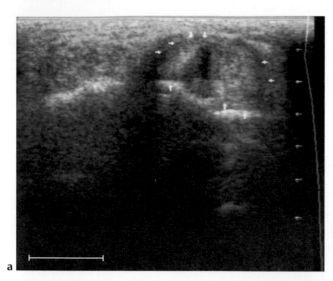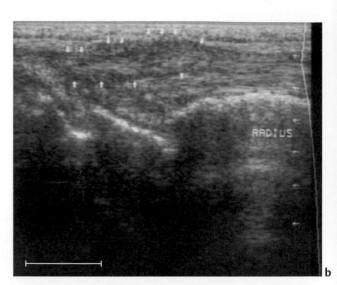

Fig. 244
Diffuse thickening of the abductor pollicis longus and extensor pollicis brevis tendons (→), with a nodular aspect, indicates amyloid infiltration in the substance of the tendon (**a** and **b**).

Amyloid deposit in the wrist typically occurs in patients with chronic renal failure who require dialysis. It is usually symmetrical, and can lead to carpal tunnel syndrome. Amyloid deposit can be found in soft tissues, joint capsule, tendon, bone, synovial membrane, and articular cartilage.

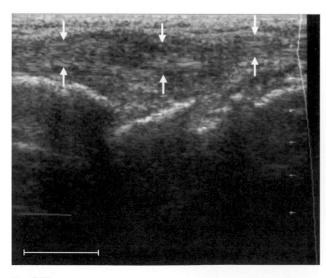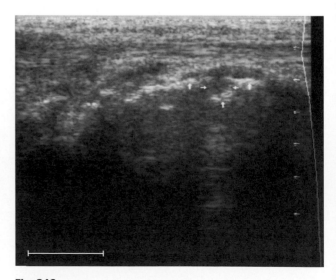

Fig. 245
Echoic infiltration of the synovial wall and of the tendon is noted in the extensor tendon (→) on this longitudinal scan.

Fig. 246
Echoic deposits are also noted on the bony surfaces causing erosions (→) on the dorsal side of the carpal bones.

Anatomy

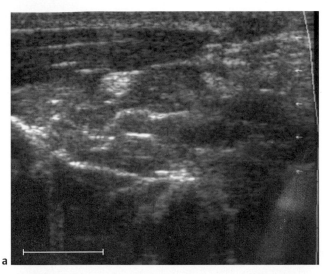
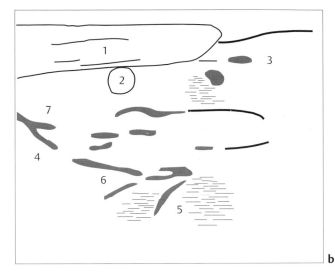

Fig. 247
Palmar transverse scan at the level of the thenar eminence. Thenar muscle (**1**), flexor pollicis longus tendon (**2**), flexor digitorum tendon (**3**), first metacarpal (**4**), second metacarpal (**5**), dorsal interosseous (**6**), abductor pollicis muscle (**7**) (**a** and **b**).

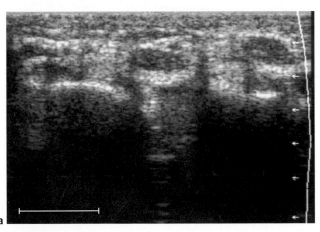
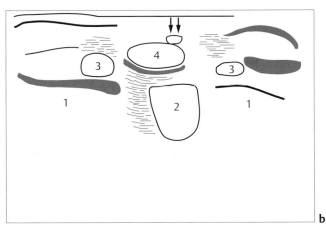

Fig. 248
Palmar transverse scan at the level of the metacarpal bones. Metacarpal bone (**1**), interosseous palmaris muscle (**2**), flexor profundus tendon (**3**), lumbricalis muscle (**4**), vessels (→) (**a** and **b**).

The longitudinal scans of the palm demonstrate the paired superficial and deep flexor tendons of the fingers. In the thenar area, the flexor pollicis longus tendon is easily identified by its marked echogenicity in comparison to the hypoechoic surrounding muscles. The tendon lies between the thenar muscles anteriorly and the adductor pollicis muscle posteriorly, the latter has a prominent muscle belly, which extends medially to the third metacarpal bone. The hypothenar, thenar, and adductor pollicis muscles are anterior to the lumbrical and interosseous muscles.

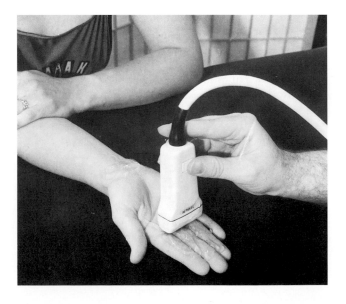

Fig. 249
Position for the anterior digital evaluation.

Hand

Anatomy

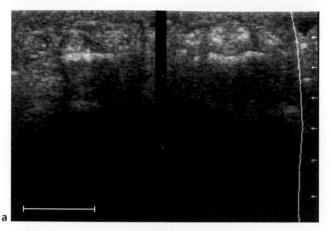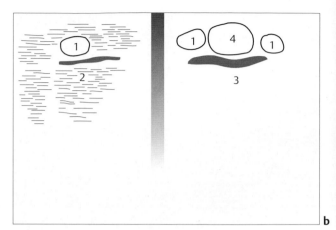

Fig. 250
Palmar transverse scan of the digits. Flexor digitorum profundus tendon (**1**), distal phalanx (**2**), proximal phalanx (**3**), flexor digitorum superficialis tendon (**4**) (**a** and **b**).

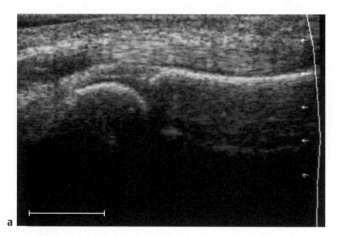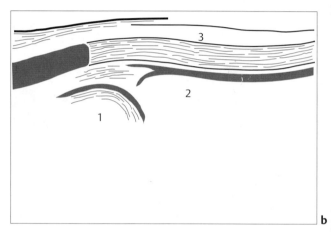

Fig. 251
Longitudinal palmar scan of the metacarpophalangeal joint. Metacarpal head (**1**), proximal phalanx (**2**), flexor digitorum superficialis tendon (**3**) (**a** and **b**).

At the metacarpal level, the cross section of the superficial and deep flexor tendons of the fingers are hyperechoic and rounded. They are adjacent to the hypoechoic lumbrical muscles. Distal to the superficial palmar arch, the cross sections of the common digital arteries are visualized, due to their pulsatile flow. The hypoechoic interosseous muscles are seen posteriorly, whereas the metacarpal bones are identified by their hyperechoic anterior cortex and acoustic shadow. With more proximal transverse scanning, the cross sections of the flexor tendons converge toward the carpal tunnel. At the phalangeal level, the flexor digitorum superficialis splits, creating a passage for the flexor digitorum profundus. It is seen as three distinct hyperechoic tendinous structures.

Anatomy

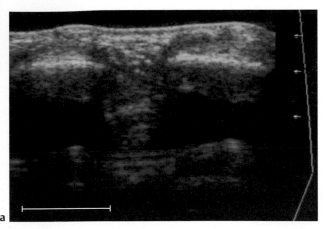
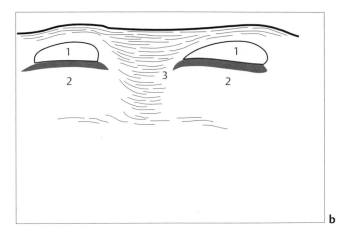

Fig. 252
Dorsal transverse scan of the metacarpal head. Extensor digitorum tendon (**1**), metacarpal head (**2**), collateral ligament (**3**) (**a** and **b**).

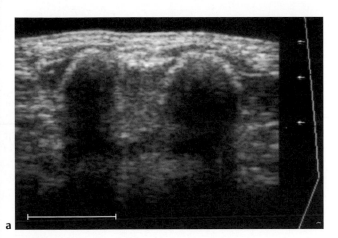
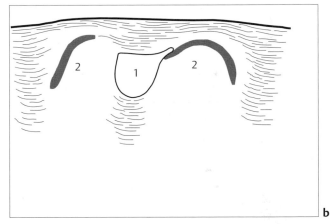

Fig. 253
Dorsal transverse scan of the metacarpal bones. Dorsal interosseous muscle (**1**), metacarpal bone (**2**) (**a** and **b**).

On the dorsal aspect of the hand and fingers, the extensor tendons, which are characterized by their fibrillar and hyperechoic texture are shown. At the posterior phalangeal level, the hyperechoic extensor expansion covers the phalangeal width. The metacarpophalangeal and interphalangeal joints are reinforced on their lateral and medial aspects by hyperechoic collateral ligaments. The medial collateral ligament of the thumb is of particular interest, as it is commonly injured. The hyaline cartilage and hypoechoic synovial membrane can be evaluated as in other synovial joints.

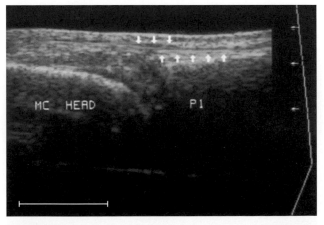

Fig. 254
Dorsal sagittal scan of the metacarpophalangeal joint. Extensor digitorum tendon (→).

Hand

Anatomy

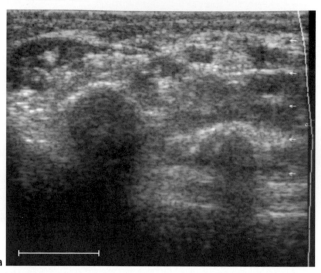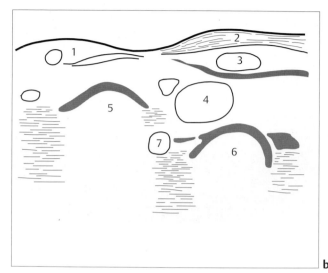

Fig. 255
Palmar transverse scan of the hypothenar. Hypothenar muscle (**1**), palmar aponeurosis (**2**), flexor digitorum muscle (**3**), palmaris brevis muscle (**4**), fifth metacarpal (**5**), fourth metacarpal (**6**) (**a** and **b**).

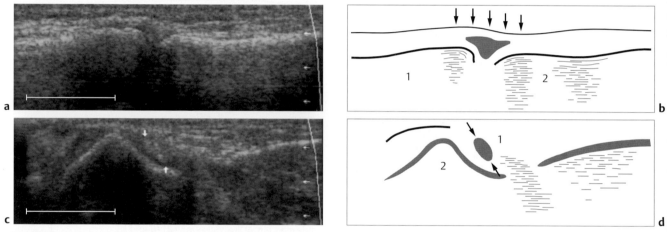

Fig. 256
Longitudinal scan of the ulnar collateral ligament of the thumb (→) (**a** and **b**). First metacarpal (**1**), first phalanx (**2**). Transverse scan of the distal first metacarpal (**c** and **d**). Ulnar collateral ligament of the thumb (**1**), first metacarpal (**2**).

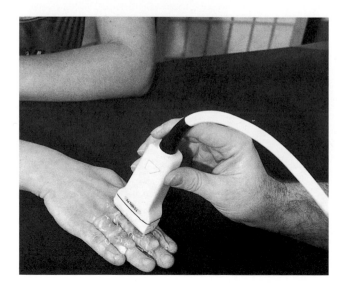

Flexor tendons can show hypoechoic segments due to their curved course and the difficulty in positioning the transducer perpendicular to their axes. Palmar and dorsal evaluation of the hand should be performed in close apposition to the fingers, filling the interdigital spaces with gel. A dynamic examination improves diagnostic capabilities.

Fig. 257
Position for a posterior digital evaluation.

Tenosynovitis

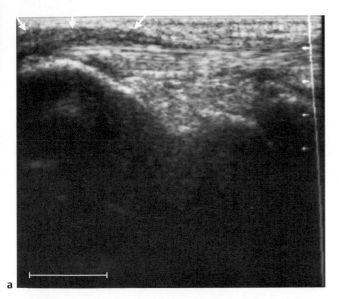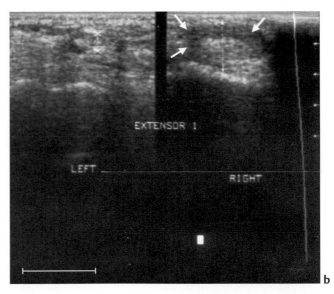

Fig. 258
Comparative longitudinal (**a**) and transverse (**b**) scans show a chronic tenosynovitis of the extensor indicis, with tendon thickening and echoic synovial thickening (→).

As flexor tendons have a synovial sheath on a great part of their course, tendinitis is accompanied by tenosynovitis. Acute and chronic tenosynovitis have the same appearance as in other locations. Tenosynovitis is best evaluated in a transverse orientation. In acute tenosynovitis, the tendon is surrounded by anechoic fluid, appearing target-like on transverse scans; the synovial membrane is not seen, or is thin. In chronic tenosynovitis, the content is more echoic and the synovium is thickened, hypoechoic, sometimes nodular as in rheumatoid arthritis. Tenosynovitis can be traumatic, inflammatory, or infectious.

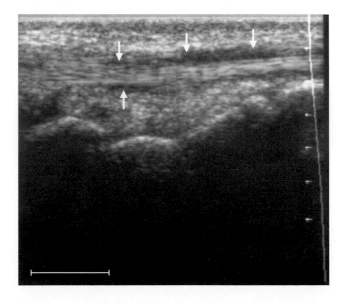

Fig. 259
A longitudinal scan of an acute tenosynovitis of the extensor of the third finger shows the tendon surrounded by hypoechoic fluid (→).

Hand

Rheumatoid Arthritis

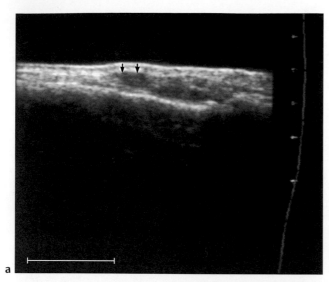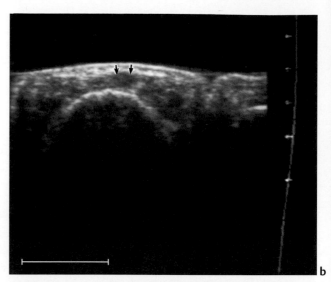

a   b

Fig. 260
Longitudinal and transverse scans of the extensor tendon of the fourth finger at the level of the second phalanx show an echoic rheumatoid nodule (→) (**a** and **b**).

In rheumatoid joints, examination of the metacarpophalangeal and the proximal interphalangeal joints can demonstrate effusion and bone erosions. The articular fluid is hypoechoic, and the bone erosions appear as irregularities of the hyperechoic cortex, which may contain a hypertrophic, echoic synovium. Lesions with their typical symmetrical distribution can be detected before they become clinically or radiologically evident. Tenosynovitis, complicated by nodules, can destroy the tendons, as shown above (p. 111).

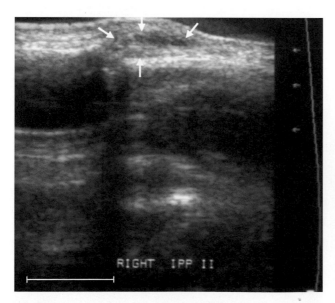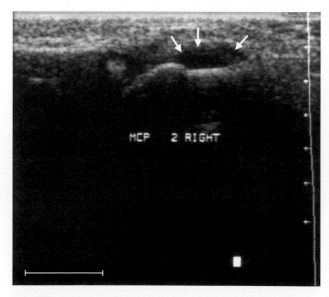

Fig. 261
Hypoechoic synovial proliferation (→) at the proximal interphalangeal joint of the second finger on a longitudinal scan.

Fig. 262
Synovial proliferation (→) and effusion is noted at the metacarpophalangeal joint of the index in a sagittal plane.

Tendon Rupture

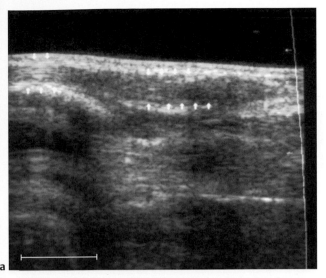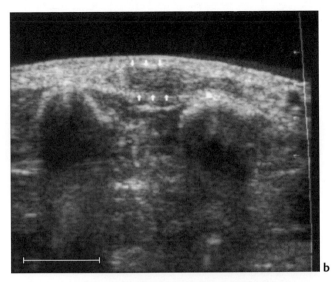

Fig. 263
Chronic rupture of the extensor indicis tendon, which has been replaced by an echoic nonfibrillar mass (→) seen in sagittal (**a**) and axial scans (→) (**b**).

Ultrasound can demonstrate tendon rupture by showing the free ends of the tendon. A hematoma or a fluid-filled sheath remains at the rupture site. In chronic cases, the tendon is replaced by echoic granulation tissue. Mallet finger results either from extensor tendon damage or from bone avulsion. Ultrasound allows distinction between a tendinous or osseous origin.

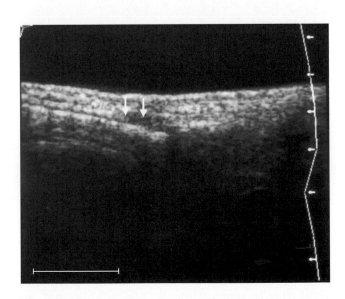

Fig. 264
Rupture of the extensor tendon (→) at the level of the distal interphalangeal joint, creating a mallet finger of tendinous origin.

Osteoarthritis

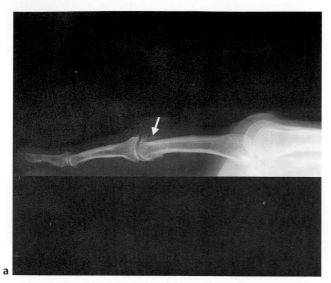
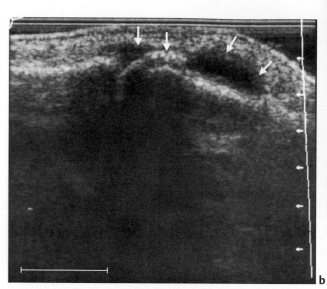

Fig. 265
An osteophyte on the metacarpal head and a capsular distension, characteristic of osteoarthritis, seen on plain film (**a**) and on ultrasound (→) (**b**).

Degenerative changes are very common in the hand, especially at the interphalangeal joints and carpometacarpal joint of the thumb. When performing ultrasound on the hand, one should be aware of the most common findings of osteoarthritis, including joint effusion with capsular distension and laxity, mucous cyst formation, cartilage destruction, and osteophyte formation.

Dupuytren's Contracture

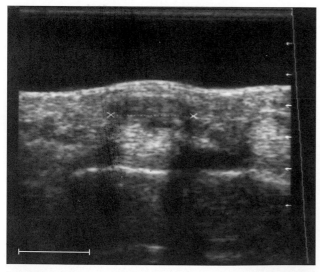
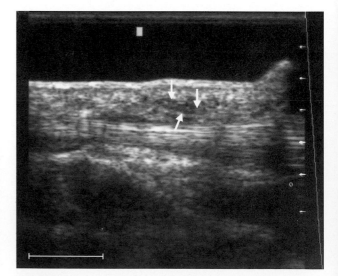

Fig. 266
A nodule (→), less echoic than the underlying flexor tendon, found in the aponeurosis at the level of the fourth metacarpal in a transverse plane.

Fig. 267
A linear echoic structure (→), found in the subcutaneous tissue at the base of the fifth finger in a sagittal plane.

Dupuytren's contracture is typically present in middle-aged and elderly men, and affects preferentially the third to fifth finger. Nodules and cords of collagen are found in the subcutaneous tissue, palmar fascia, or aponeurosis. Ultrasound detects and localizes the lesions.

Tenosynovial Cyst

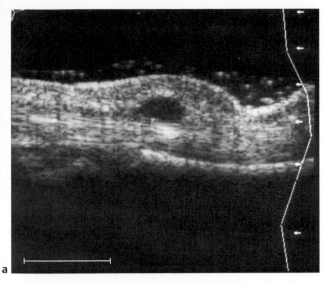 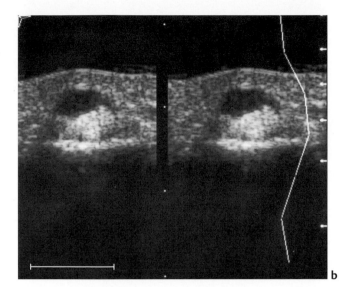

a

b

Fig. 268
An anechoic tenosynovial cyst in a longitudinal and transverse plane (**a** and **b**).

Synovial cysts may arise from synovial sheaths, and appear as anechoic masses, usually of round or oval shape, communicating with a synovial sheath. Clinically, a tender and painful small mass is present.

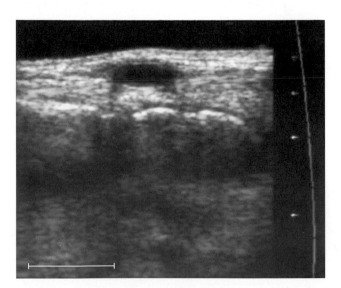

Fig. 269
An anechoic cyst of the extensor tendon sheath, seen on a sagittal image.

Hand

Gamekeeper's Thumb

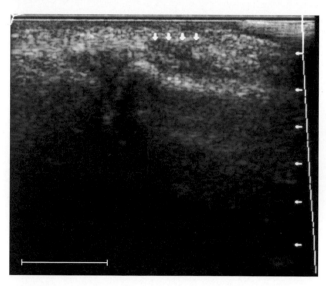

Fig. 270
A longitudinal scan of the metacarpophalangeal joint shows the interrupted ligament and the free ends separated by an hypoechoic zone (→).

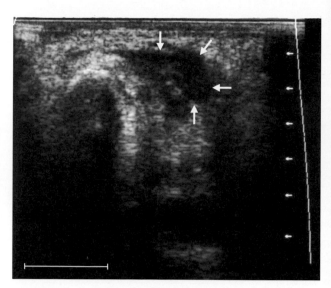

Fig. 271
In a transverse approach, a hypoechoic mass (→) is seen medial to the metacarpal head and the overlying extensor tendon, corresponding to a Stener's lesion.

Gamekeeper's thumb is a rupture of the ulnar collateral ligament of the thumb. This lesion is a frequent skiing injury. If the ruptured ligament is displaced and uncovered by the aponeurosis (Stener's lesion), surgery is required. On a transverse scan, a hypoechoic mass is seen adjacent to the metatarsal head. The hypoechoic mass, which may contain a hyperechoic center, lies between the interosseous dorsalis muscle and the metacarpal head, over the adductor policis muscle. Capsuloligamentous lesions at other sites manifest as hypoechoic swellings. Pathological joint laxity can be demonstrated by ultrasound.

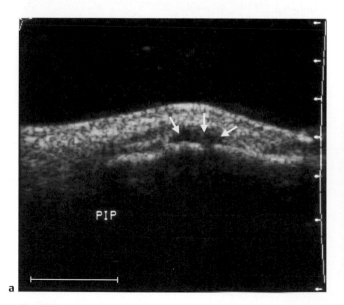

Fig. 272
A hypoechoic swelling (→) at the interphalangeal joint of the thumb after trauma (**a**). Pathological distension (→) is noted on stress (**b**).

Normal and Pathologic Regional Ultrasound Lower Extremities

Hip

Thigh

Knee

Leg

Ankle

Foot

Infant Hip

Anatomy

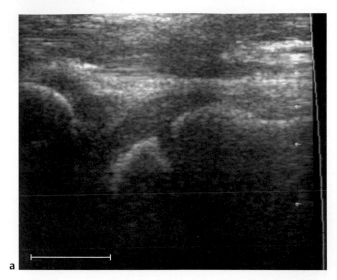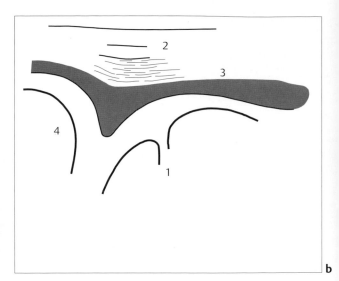

Fig. 273
Parasagittal scan. Growth plate (**1**), psoas muscle (**2**), iliofemoral ligament and joint capsule (**3**), acetabulum (**4**) (**a** and **b**).

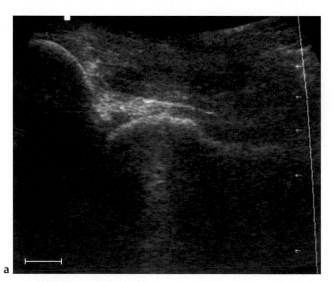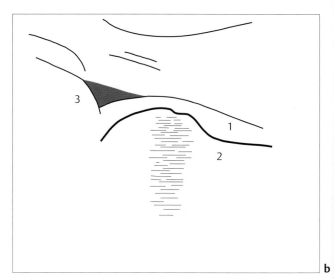

Fig. 274
Parasagittal scan. Anterior recess (**1**), femoral neck (**2**), acetabulum (**3**) (**a** and **b**).

The parasagittal plane of the hip is obtained parallel to the femoral neck with the femur and knee in extension and external rotation. The normal cartilaginous femoral head is spherical, with a diameter of 1cm in the neonate to 2cm at 6 months of age. It contains fine hyperechoic dots, presumably due to vascularity. A small ossification center of the femoral head can be discerned before it becomes visible on radiographs. If large, this ossification center can obscure the acetabu-lum. The hypoechoic cartilaginous greater trochanter is continuous with the cartilaginous head and neck on transverse and coronal scans. The cartilaginous greater trochanter should be recognized as a hypo-echoic structure near the cartilaginous head and neck on transverse and coronal scans. The bony acetabu-lum is covered by a hypoechoic hyaline cartilage and prolonged at its outer border by the hyperechoic trian-gular labrum.

Anatomy

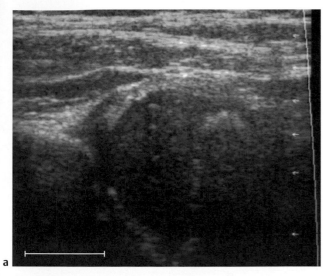
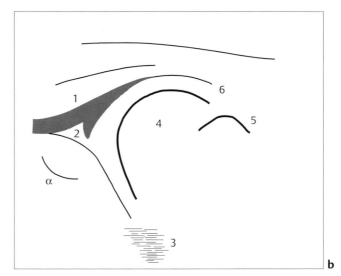

Fig. 275
Coronal plane of the left hip in a 4-month-old child, in a supine position, the hip slighty flexed and internally rotated. Labrum (**1**), hyaline cartilage of acetabular roof (**2**), vertical portion of the triradiate cartilage (**3**), femoral head (**4**), greater trochanter (**5**), joint capsule (**6**) (**a** and **b**).

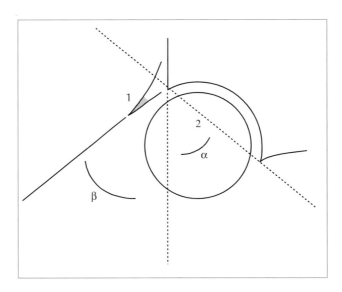

Fig. 276
Echogenic acetabular labrum (**1**), femoral head (**2**), measurement of α and β angle.

The triradiate hypoechoic cartilage connects the inferior border of the acetabulum to the pubic and ischial bone centers. The hyperechoic iliofemoral ligament forms the anterior joint capsule (well seen in a sagittal plane), and is used as a landmark for the evaluation of the anterior recess. Flexion of the hip to 45 degrees decompresses the anterior recess and can simulate hip effusion. Comparative measurements of the thickness of the hypoechoic proximal femoral growth plate is useful in the diagnosis of epiphysiolysis. Two techniques are used to evaluate the position of the femoral head. The technique of Graf uses a coronal plane to determine the percentage of coverage of the femoral head. The alpha angle is the angle between the tangent line of the acetabular concavity and the tangent line of the anterior edge of the bony acetabulum and measures the "osseous acetabulum."

Infant Hip

Anatomy

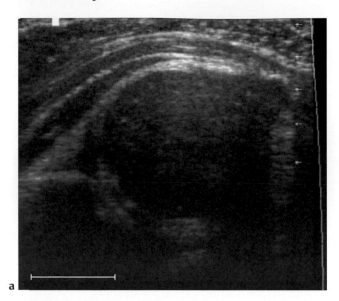
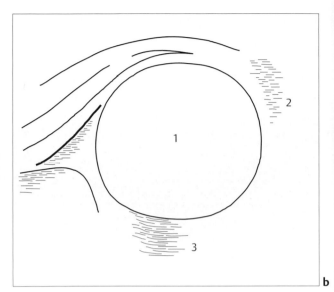

Fig. 277
Lateral transverse view of the flexed hip. Femoral head (**1**), greater trochanter (**2**), triradiate cartilage (**3**) (**a** and **b**).

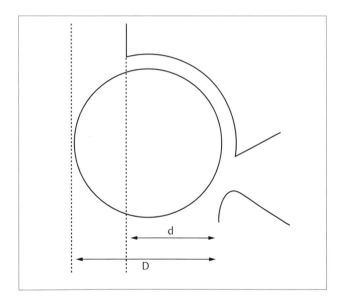

Fig. 278
Lateral transverse view of the flexed hip. Head coverage and head size measurement. Ratio d/D represents percentage of coverage.

A small alpha angle indicates a dysplasia of acetabulum. The beta angle is measured between the anterior edge of the bony acetabulum and the line tangent to the labrum. It gives an indication of coverage of the femoral head by the labrum. A large beta angle indicates lateral migration of the femoral head. The technique of Harcke uses transverse planes with the femur at 90 degrees of flexion and evaluates the stability of the hip by pushing down on the flexed knee, similar to the clinical examination. Echoes from the bony acetabulum appear posterior to the femoral head and produce a U configuration in the normal hip, with the triradiate cartilage bisecting the femoral head. With this method, a ratio of femoral head coverage can be measured.

Anatomy

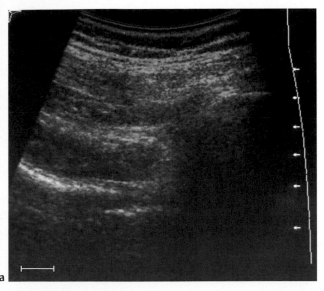
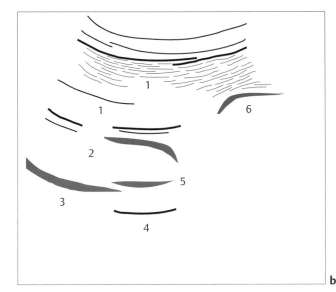

Fig. 279
Coronal view at the level of the greater trochanter. Gluteus medius (**1**), gluteus minimus muscle (**2**), acetabulum (**3**), femoral head (**4**), ilio-femoral ligament (**5**), greater trochanter (**6**) (**a** and **b**).

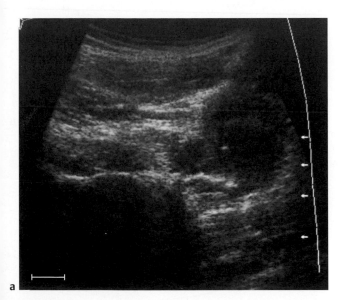
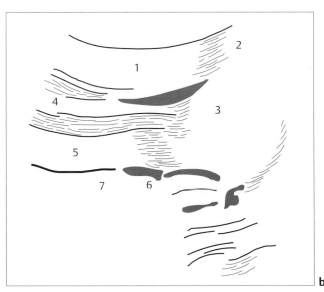

Fig. 280
Midcoronal view of the hip joint. Tensor fasciae latae (**1**), rectus femoris (**2**), iliopsoas (**3**), gluteus medius (**4**), gluteus minimus (**5**) muscles, iliofemoral ligament (**6**), femoral head (**7**) (**a** and **b**).

The gluteus medius and tensor fasciae latae muscles form the superficial muscles lying proximal and distal to the greater trochanter in a coronal view. The gluteus minimus muscle lies between the gluteus medius muscle and the hyperechoic iliofemoral ligament covering the femoral neck. The vastus lateralis muscle is situated deep to the tensor fasciae latae muscle. Imaging of the femoral head and neck in an anterior transverse plane depicts the femoral vein, artery, and nerve from medial to lateral, situated anterior to the iliopsoas muscle and tendon.

Hip

Anatomy

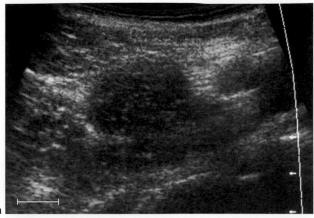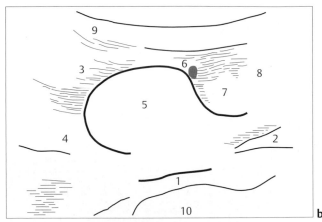

Fig. 281
Medial transverse view of the hip joint by an anterior approach. Iliofemoral ligament (**1**), labrum (**2**), rectus femoris tendon (**3**), gluteus minimus (**4**), iliopsoas (**5**) muscles, femoral nerve (**6**), lateral femoral circumflex artery (**7**), vein (**8**), sartorius muscle (**9**), femoral head (**10**) (**a** and **b**).

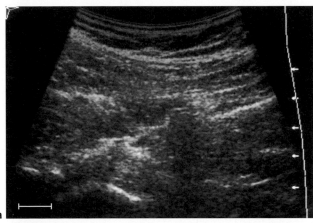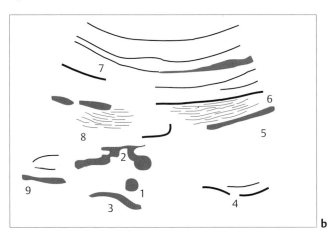

Fig. 282
Lateral transverse view at the level of the acetabular labrum. Iliofemoral ligament (**1**), rectus femoris muscle tendon (**2**), femoral head (**3**), iliopsoas (**4**), rectus femoris muscle (**5**), fasciae latae (**6**), tensor fasciae latae (**7**), gluteus minimus (**8**) muscles, acetabulum (**9**) (**a** and **b**).

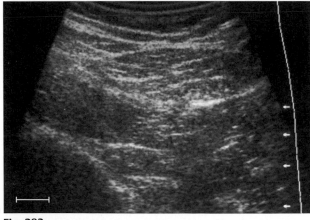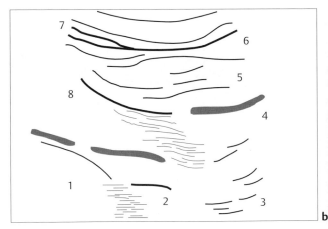

Fig. 283
Inferior transverse view by a lateral approach. Femur (**1**), iliopsoas (**2**), adductor (**3**), pectineus (**4**), rectus femoris (**5**), sartorius (**6**), tensor fasciae latae (**7**), vastus lateralis (**8**) muscles (**a** and **b**).

The tensor fasciae latae muscle and the deeper gluteus medius muscle have a superficial and a more posterior location seen on an anterolateral approach. The gluteus minimus muscle lies between these two muscles and the hyperechoic ilio-femoral ligament. Medial to the femoral vessels, the pectineus and the more posterior located obturator externus muscles can be found.

Anatomy

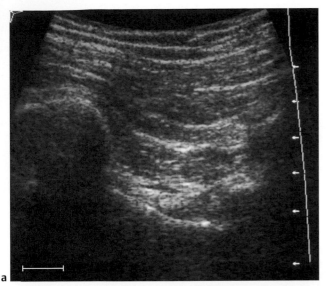
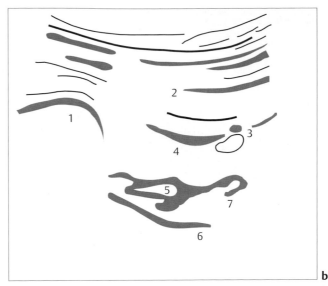

Fig. 284
Transverse view at the hip joint by a posterior approach. Greater trochanter (**1**), gluteus maximus muscle (**2**), sciatic nerve (**3**), inferior gemellus muscle (**4**), ischiofemoral ligament (**5**), femoral head (**6**), acetabulum (**7**) (**a** and **b**).

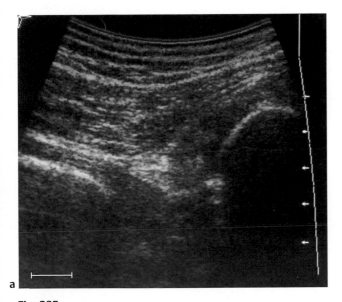
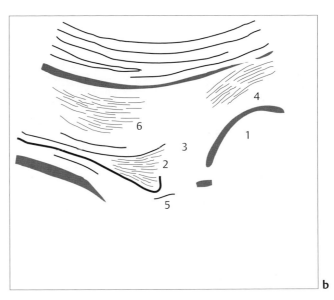

Fig. 285
Transverse view at the level of the insertion of the hamstrings by a posterior approach. Ischium (**1**), sciatic nerve (**2**), semimembranosus (**3**), biceps femoris and semitendinosus tendons (**4**), quadratus femoris (**5**), gluteus maximus (**6**) muscles (**a** and **b**).

In posterior transverse scans, the gluteus maximus muscle covers from lateral to medial the gluteus medius muscle, the greater trochanter, the inferior gemellus muscle in a proximal plane, and the quadratus femoris muscle in a more caudal plane. More distally, the gluteus maximus muscle covers the ischium with the inserting hamstring tendons. The sciatic nerve is a thick hyperechoic fibrillar structure easily found between the gluteus maximus muscle posteriorly, the quadratus femoris muscle anteriorly, and the ischium and the semimembranosus tendon insertion laterally. The semimembranosus tendon inserts on the posterolateral border of the ischium, the biceps femoris and semitendinosus tendons are inseparable at their insertion on the posterior border of the ischium. These three hamstring tendons often appear hypoechoic at their insertion and should be evaluated by a comparative study.

Anatomy

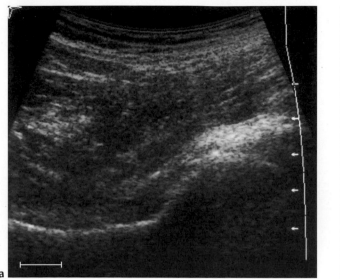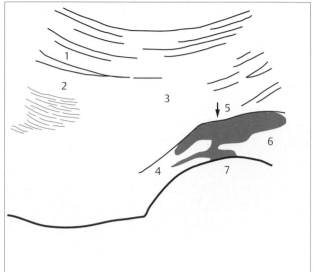

Fig. 286
Lateral sagittal view by an anterior approach. Sartorius (**1**), rectus femoris (**2**), iliopsoas (**3**) muscles, iliofemoral ligament (**4**), rectus femoris tendon (**5**), acetabulum (**6**), femoral head (**7**) (**a** and **b**).

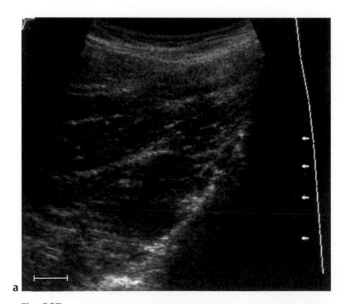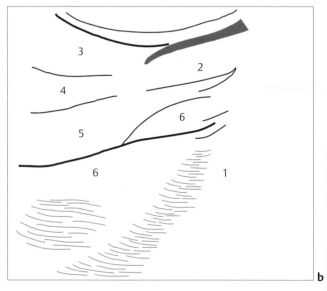

Fig. 287
Medial sagittal view by an anterior approach. Pubis (**1**), pectineus (**2**), adductor longus (**3**), adductor brevis (**4**), adductor magnus (**5**), obturator externus (**6**) muscles (**a** and **b**).

The joint capsule can be seen as a concave linear echoic structure extending from the acetabular ring to its insertion on the peritrochanteric region of the femur and is composed by the iliofemoral ligament anteriorly and the ischiofemoral ligament posteriorly. These ligaments cover the anterior and posterior labrum. They are seen as hyperechoic cartilaginous triangles, extending from the acetabular margins.

Anatomy

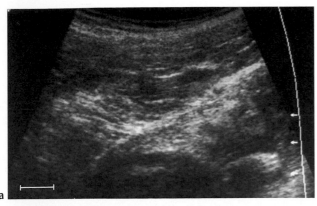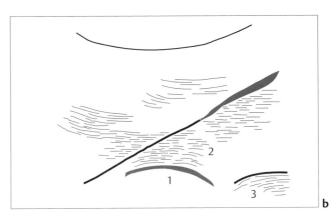

Fig. 288
Sagittal view of the hip joint by an anterior approach. Femoral head (**1**), labrum (**2**), acetabulum (**3**) (**a** and **b**).

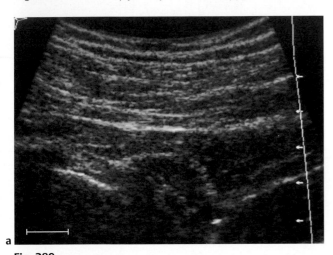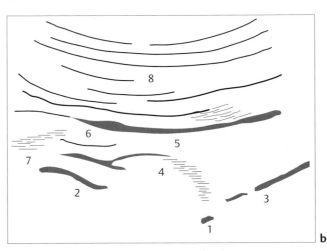

Fig. 289
Mid sagittal view by a posterior approach. Mediofemoral circumflex artery (**1**), femur (**2**), adductor (**3**), obturator externus (**4**), quadratus femoris (**5**), gemellus (**6**) muscles, acetabulum (**7**), gluteus maximus muscle (**8**) (**a** and **b**).

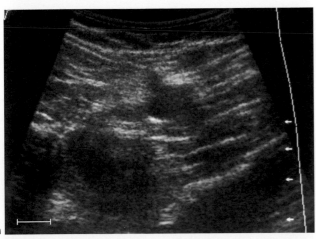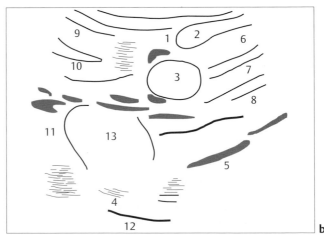

Fig. 290
Inferior transverse view by an anterior approach. Femoral nerve (**1**), superficial femoral vessels (**2**), deep femoral vessels (**3**), iliofemoral ligament (**4**), quadratus femoris (**5**), pectineus (**6**), adductor longus (**7**), adductor brevis (**8**), sartorius (**9**), rectus femoris (**10**), vastus lateralis (**11**) muscles, femur (**12**), iliopsoas muscle and tendon (**13**) (**a** and **b**).

In a more lateral sagittal plane, the insertion of the rectus femoris tendon can be seen on the anteroinferior iliac spine. In a more medial sagittal plane, the adductor muscles are seen, composed of the adductor longus, brevis and magnus muscles from anterior to posterior.

Hip

Effusion

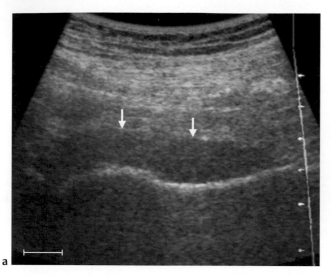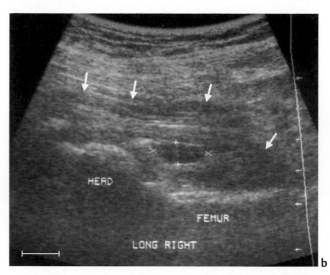

Fig. 291
This effusion (→) is homogeneously filled with small echoes. Puncture confirmed the diagnosis of septic arthritis (**a**). Another septic arthritis with a hypoechoic content (→) is shown and a small abscess is disclosed. Note also the bone irregularities of the femoral head (**b**).

In case of effusion, the hyperechoic iliofemoral ligament is displaced from the femoral neck by a hypoechoic or anechoic band. Ultrasound is sensitive for detection of effusion, but is not specific. In infections, the effusion is hypoechoic, rich in tiny echoes, ending up in a hyperechoic appearance, similar to the echogenicity of muscles in selected cases. Aspiration can be performed under sonographic control. In inflammatory disorders, the contents are also hypoechoic, and the effusion is often bilateral, as in rheumatoid arthritis.

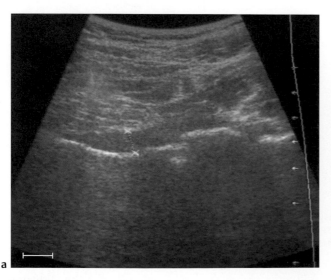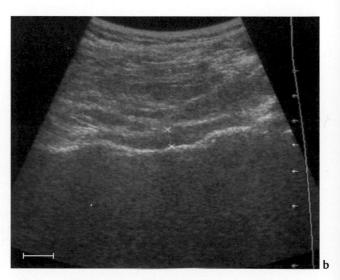

Fig. 292
Bilateral synovial thickening is seen in this patient with rheumatoid arthritis. The reaction predominates on the side on which bone erosion is observed (**a** and **b**).

Effusions in Children

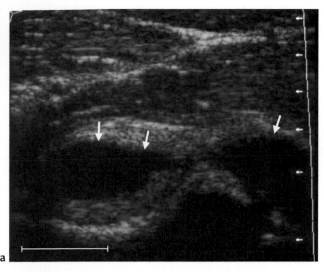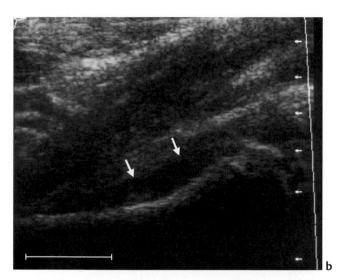

Fig. 293
Hip effusions (→) of various amounts demonstrated in a sagittal plane in infants with transient synovitis (**a** and **b**).

The most common cause of effusion in children is transient synovitis. The diagnosis is confirmed by the resolution of the effusion in two or three weeks. Otherwise, a Legg–Calve–Perthes disease is suspected. In advanced cases of Legg–Calve–Perthes disease, the epiphysis is deformed. In infections, the effusion appears more echoic and clinical evolution is fulminant.

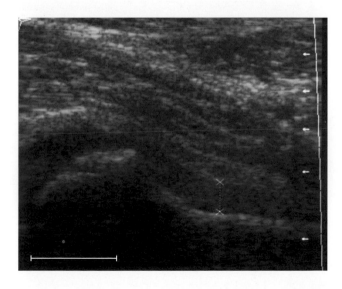

Fig. 294
Legg–Calve–Perthes disease with deformed epiphysis and a small hip effusion.

Hip

Bursitis

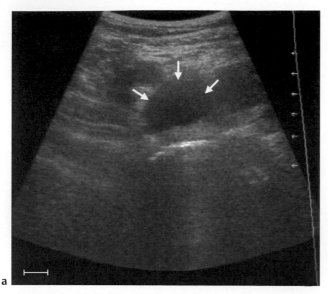
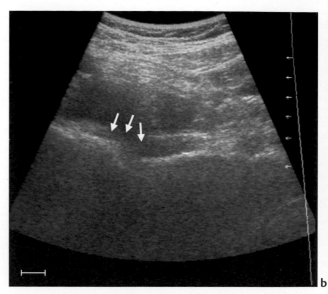

Fig. 295
An iliopsoas bursitis appears as an almost anechoic cyst-like lesion on a transverse scan, interposed between the femoral vessels and the iliopsoas muscle, in this patient, who experienced a snapping sensation in the hip (**a**). The longitudinal scan shows the location of the bursitis deep to the iliopsoas muscle and its communication (→) with the coxofemoral joint (**b**).

Trochanteric bursitis or iliopsoas bursitis can cause hip pain. A communication between the iliopsoas bursa and the hip joint is present in 20% of adults. Trochanteric bursitis is mainly caused by friction, but specific etiologies, such as tuberculosis, must be searched for. Ultrasound will show heterogeneous fluid collections, as in other infections.

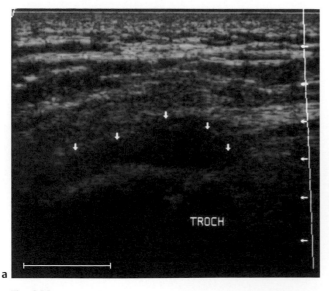
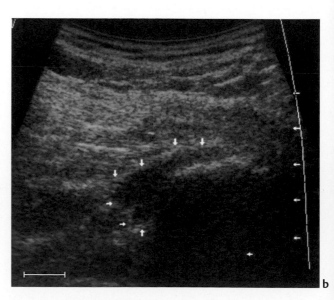

Fig. 296
Trochanteric bursitis (→) is present deep to the tensor fasciae latae at the lateroinferior border of the greater trochanter in these two patients (**a** and **b**).

Tendinitis

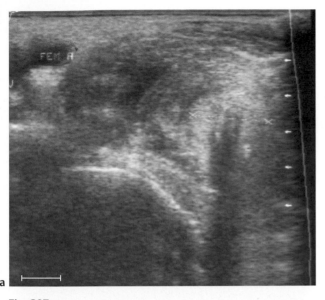
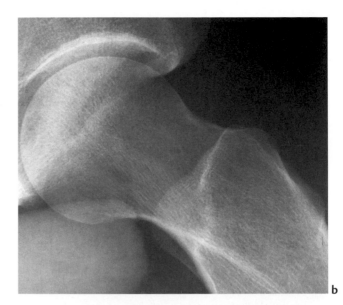

Fig. 297
A thickened rectus femoris tendon, containing calcifications and situated lateral to the iliopsoas muscle and posterior to the sartorius muscle, is shown (**a**). The corresponding plain film reveals small calcium deposits at the insertion site of the rectus femoris tendon (**b**).

Calcified tendinitis can be seen at the insertion of the gluteal muscles, and less frequently in other tendons, such as the rectus femoris muscle. Cases of tendinitis caused by hydroxyapatite cristal deposit tend to be painful, due to a severe inflammatory reaction, which can destroy the calcifications. On ultrasound, the tendon appears swollen, sometimes hypoechoic, and contains hyperechoic deposits, with or without an acoustic shadow.

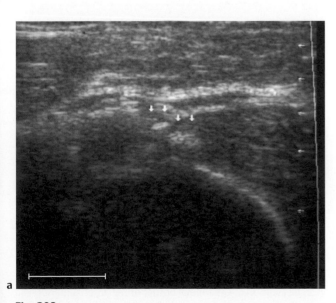
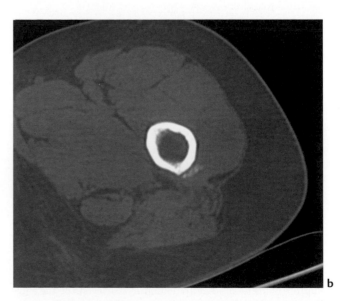

Fig. 298
Calcifications of the gluteus maximus muscle near its insertion on the posterior aspect of the femur (**a**). CT of the same patient confirms the calcifications (**b**).

Hip

Sports Injuries

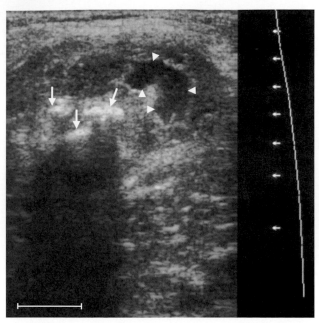

Fig. 299
An anechoic collection (▶) as a sign of partial rupture of the adductor longus muscle. Calcifications as sequelae (→) of repetitive trauma.

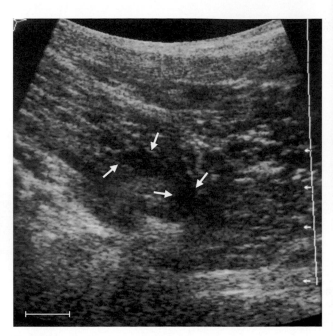

Fig. 300
This ballet dancer felt a sudden pain in the medial aspect of the thigh on exercise. Ultrasound revealed a partial tear (→) of the adductor brevis muscle (oblique transverse scan).

Muscular and enthesis trauma in the pelvis and particularly the hip are frequently observed in sports. Adductor muscles are prone to repetitive trauma in dancers, horse riders, and soccer players. Pain in the symphysis pubis is frequent in marathon runners and soccer players. Degenerative changes can occur, but also anterior symphyseal instability, which can be evaluated on ultrasound when the patient stands on one foot.

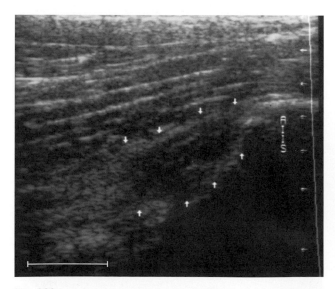

Fig. 301
Rupture of the rectus femoris tendon at its insertion on the anteroinferior iliac spine is shown as an anechoic gap (→). The sartorius muscle is overlying the lesion.

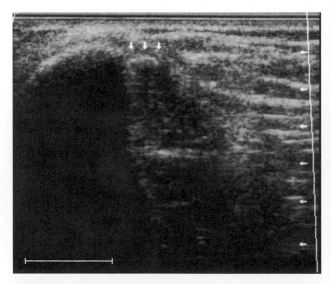

Fig. 302
A small avulsion at the medial border of the anterosuperior iliac spine (→) not seen on a plain film, and which occurred after exercising the abdominal muscles. It corresponds to the insertion site of the oblique abdominal muscles.

Hamstring Tendinitis

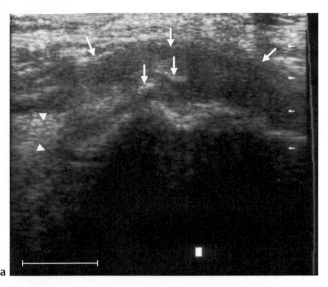 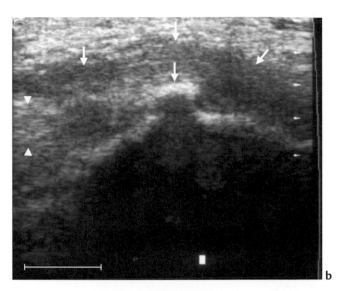

Fig. 303
Examples of hamstring tendinitis in two patients show thickening, calcifications (→) (**a**), and bone irregularities (**b**). Notice the hyperechoic sciatic nerve (▶) lateral to the semimembranosus tendon.

The semimembranosus tendon inserts on the posterolateral edge of the ischium. The biceps femoris and semitendinosus tendon are seen as a single tendon insertion on the posteromedial ischial border. Tendinitis should be evaluated by a comparative axial study of the tendon insertion. Thickening and a hypoechoic appearance are positive signs of inflammation. Calcifications can be seen, and appear as hyperechoic foci, with or without an acoustic shadow. Bone irregularities can also be observed.

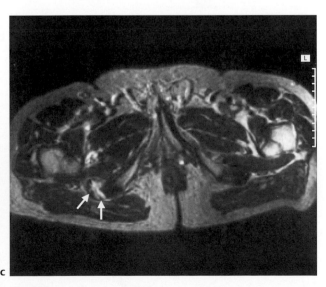 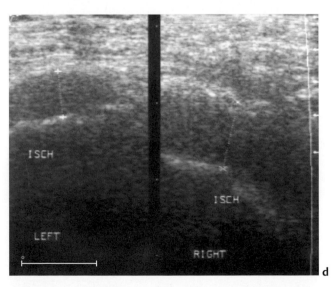

Fig. 303
MRI of the patient in (**b**) shows a hyperintense signal in the hamstring tendons (→) on a T$_2$-weighted image (**c**). An asymmetrical thickening of the hamstring tendons appears on this comparative study (**d**).

Thigh

Anatomy

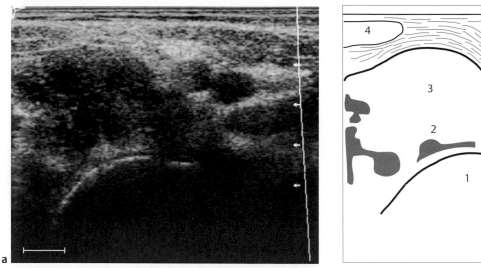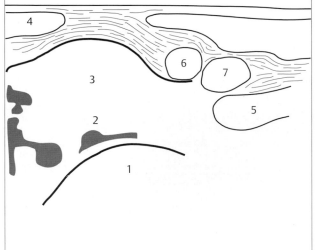

Fig. 304
Anterior transverse scan of the proximal third. Femoral head (**1**), iliopsoas tendon (**2**), iliopsoas (**3**), sartorius (**4**), pectineus (**5**) muscles, femoral artery (**6**), femoral vein (**7**) (**a** and **b**).

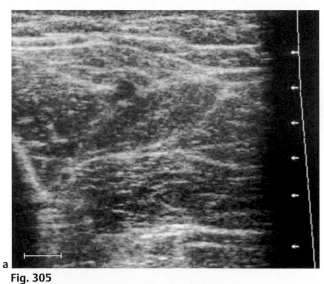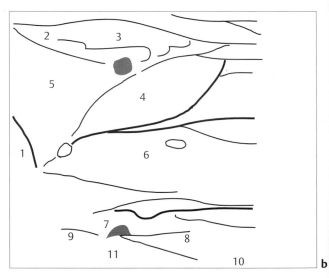

Fig. 305
Anterior transverse scan of the proximal third, medial to the femur. Femur (**1**), rectus femoris (**2**), sartorius (**3**), adductor longus (**4**), vastus medialis (**5**), adductor brevis (**6**) muscles, sciatic nerve (**7**), adductor magnus (**8**), iliopsoas (**9**), semitendinosus (**10**), biceps femoris (**11**) muscles (**a** and **b**).

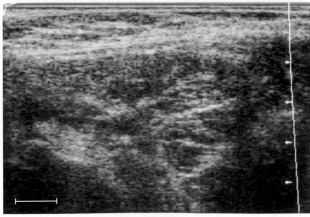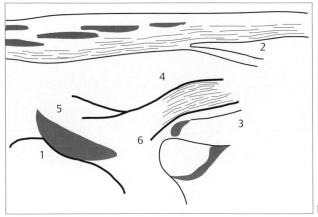

Fig. 306
Anterior transverse scan at the level of the greater trochanter. Greater trochanter (**1**), sartorius (**2**), rectus femoris (**3**), tensor fasciae latae (**4**), gluteus minimus (**5**), gluteus medius (**6**) muscles (**a** and **b**).

Anatomy

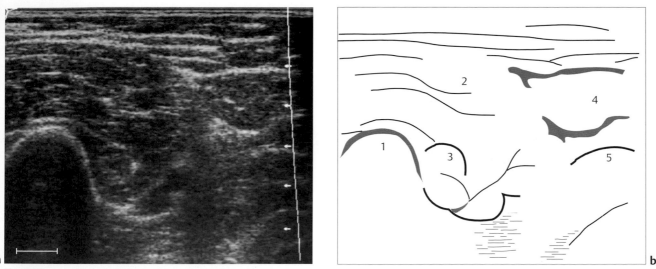

Fig. 307
Anterior medial transverse scan of the middle third. Femur (**1**), vastus medialis (**2**), vastus intermedius (**3**), sartorius (**4**), adductor longus (**5**) muscles (**a** and **b**).

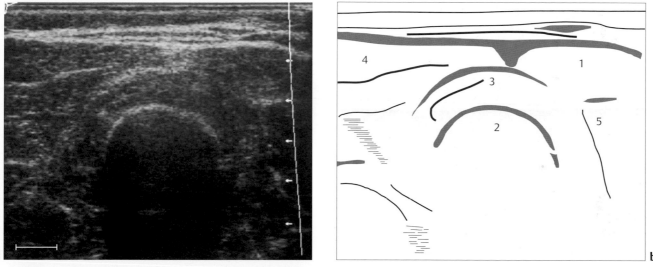

Fig. 308
Anterior lateral transverse scan of the middle third. Rectus femoris (**1**), femur (**2**), vastus intermedius (**3**), vastus lateralis (**4**), vastus medialis (**5**) muscles (**a** and **b**).

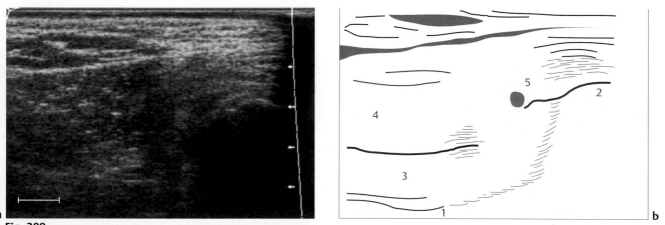

Fig. 309
Postero-lateral transverse scan of the proximal third. Femoral neck (**1**), ischium (**2**), gemellus inferior (**3**), gluteus magnus (**4**) muscles, sciatic nerve (**5**) (**a** and **b**).

Thigh

Anatomy

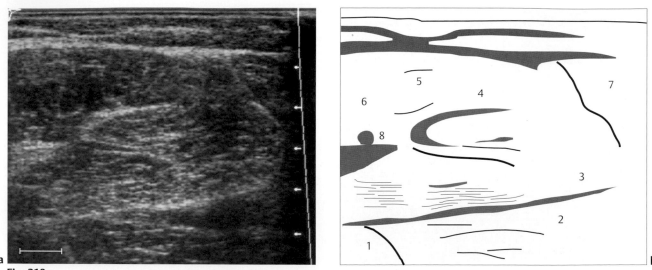

Fig. 310
Transverse scan of the posteromedial middle third. Femur (**1**), adductor longus (**2**), adductor magnus (**3**), semimembranosus (**4**), semitendinosus (**5**), biceps femoris (**6**), vastus medialis (**7**) muscles, sciatic nerve (**8**) (**a** and **b**).

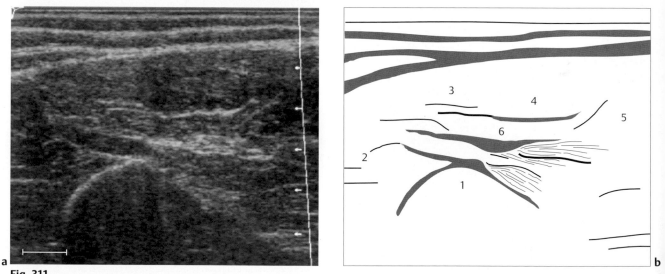

Fig. 311
Transverse scan of the posterolateral middle third. Femur (**1**), vastus lateralis (**2**), biceps femoris (**3**), semitendinosus (**4**), semimembranosus (**5**) muscle, sciatic nerve (**6**) (**a** and **b**).

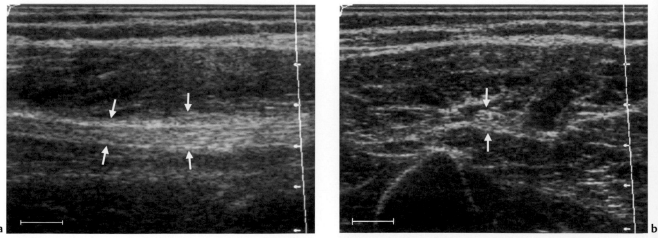

Fig. 312
Sciatic nerve (→) on a longitudinal (**a**) and transverse (**b**) view.

Anatomy

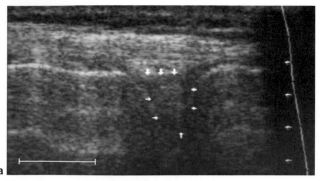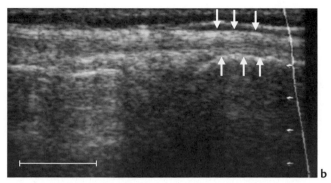

Fig. 313
Longitudinal scan of the hyperechoic medial meniscus (→) (**a**) and the medial collateral ligament (**b**), with its deep (→) and superficial portion (▶) (**a** and **b**).

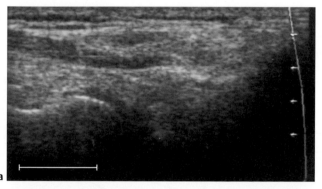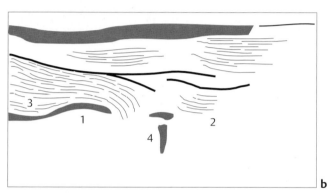

Fig. 314
Longitudinal scan. Femur (**1**), tibia (**2**), popliteus tendon (**3**), lateral meniscus (**4**) (**a** and **b**).

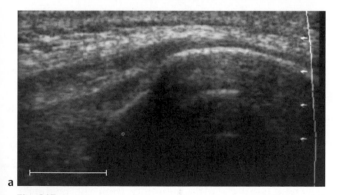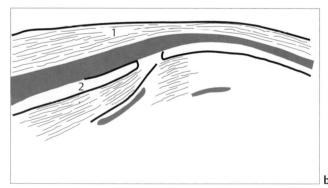

Fig. 315
Longitudinal scan of the quadriceps tendon. Rectus femoris (**1**), vastus intermedius (**2**) muscles (**a** and **b**).

The quadriceps tendon is large, superficial, and well defined due to the surrounding fat and soft tissue. The vastus medialis muscle extends to the proximal medial border of the patella, giving a broad tendon that inserts more distally on the medial border of the patella and the centromedial border of the medial femoral condyle. This structure is continued distally by the hyperechoic medial patellar retinaculum. At the external border of the patella, the hyperechoic lateral patellar retinaculum is found anterior to the tendon of the vastus lateralis muscle and the iliotibial tract, which lies on the prominent outer border of the lateral

femoral condyle. The normal menisci appear as homogeneous hyperechoic triangular structures, with the apex of the triangle pointing toward the middle of the joint. The posterior parts and outer borders of the menisci can be evaluated. The defect in the posterior horn of the lateral meniscus is created by the hyperechoic popliteus tendon. Its surrounding hypoechoic sheath has an articular communication. This tendon inserts on the corresponding fossa of the lateral femoral condyle. The bone surfaces of the femoral condyles and tibial plateaus are easily defined as highly echoic lines with acoustic shadowing.

Knee

Anatomy

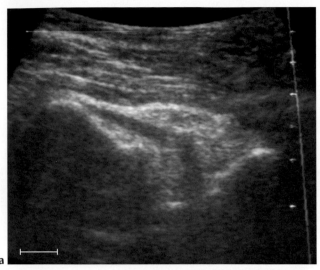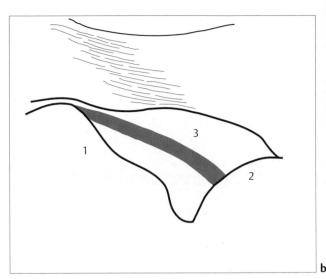

a   b

Fig. 316
Intercondylar longitudinal scan showing the posterior cruciate ligament as a hypoechoic band (**1**), tibia (**2**), femur (**3**) (**a** and **b**).

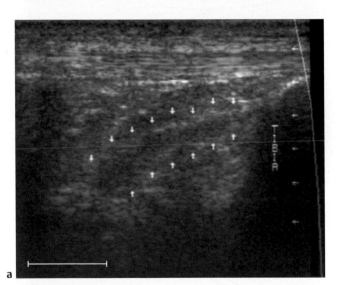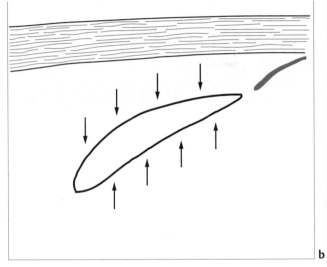

a   b

Fig. 317
The anterior cruciate ligament (→) by an anterior approach the knee flexed at 60° (**a** and **b**).

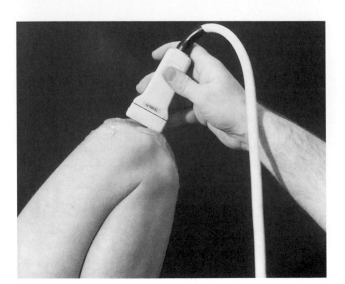

The posterior cruciate ligament can be seen as a hypoechoic band running obliquely from the posterior tibial spine to the lateral margin of the medial condyle. The hypoechoic anterior cruciate ligament is seen underneath the patella by an oblique sagittal anterior approach, the knee being flexed at least at 60°. The ligament runs obliquely from the medial margin of the lateral femoral condyle to the anterior tibial spine.

Fig. 318
Position for the evaluation of the anterior cruciate ligament and the trochlear cartilage.

Anatomy

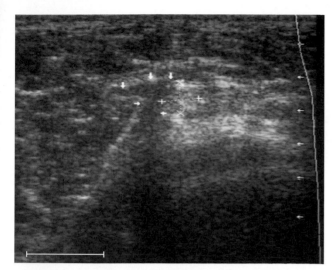

Fig. 319
Gastrocnemius-semimembranosus bursa (→).

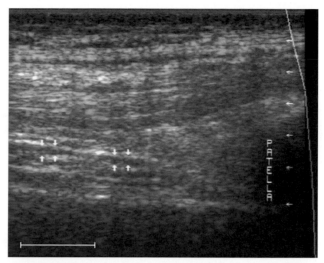

Fig. 320
Suprapatellar bursa (→).

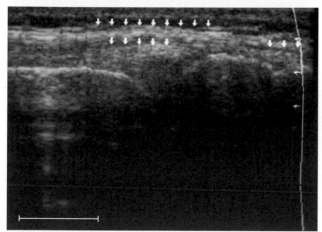

Fig. 321
Longitudinal scan of the medial collateral ligament (→).

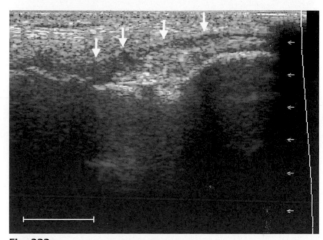

Fig. 322
Longitudinal scan of the lateral collateral ligament (→).

The gastrocnemius-semimembranosus and suprapatellar bursae are seen as hypoechoic bands, even when there is no abnormal articular distension. The semitendinosus tendon lies posterior to the semimembranosus muscle and tendon and forms with the gracilis and sartorius tendons the pes anserinus, inserting in this order from posterior to anterior on the medial cortex of the proximal tibial metaphysis. The popliteal vessels and the tibial nerve separate the medial and lateral heads of the gastrocnemius muscle. The medial collateral ligament consists of two broad parrallel hyperechoic bands, separated by hypoechoic loose areolar tissue. The deep portion inserts into the meniscus, the superficial layer inserts posteriorly into the lateral aspect of the medial tibial metaphysis and into the proximal part of the medial femoral condyle. Two structures insert into the fibular head: the thin and relatively hypoechoic lateral collateral ligament with an anterior oblique course toward the external femoral condyle, and the hyperechoic biceps femoris tendon with its oblique posterior direction. The com-

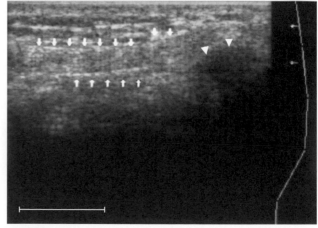

Fig. 323
Longitudinal scan of the biceps femoris tendon (→) inserting on the fibular head (▶).

mon peroneal nerve is situated posterior to the biceps tendon and lateral to the lateral head of the gastrocnemius, the plantaris, and soleus muscles.

Knee

Anatomy

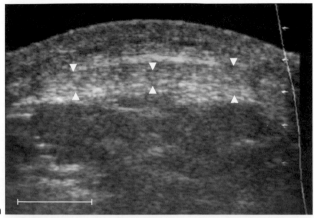
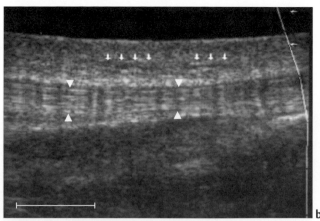

Fig. 324
Transverse (**a**) and longitudinal scan (**b**) of the patellar tendon (▶) and the prepatellar bursa (→).

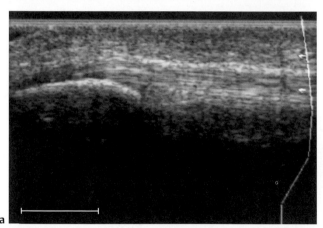
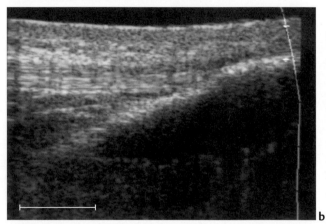

Fig. 325
Longitudinal scan of the proximal (**a**) and distal (**b**) insertion of the patellar tendon.

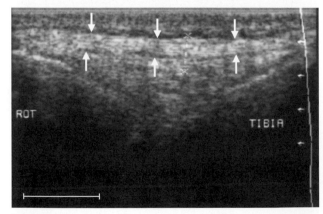
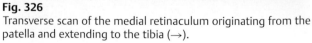

Fig. 326
Transverse scan of the medial retinaculum originating from the patella and extending to the tibia (→).

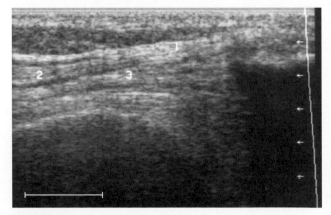

Fig. 327
Transverse antero-lateral approach of the femoro-patellar joint. Lateral retinaculum (**1**) vastus lateralis tendon (**3**), iliotibial tract (**2**).

The patellar tendon originates from the inferior border of the patella. It is widest at its origin, and narrows toward the distal insertion on the anterior tibial tuberosity. The patient is examined in a supine position, the knee slightly flexed. Comparison with the contralateral side is useful because of normal vari-

ants. The images are obtained in longitudinal and transverse planes. The normal tendon is less echoic at both insertions. The infrapatellar fat body is hypoechoic. The scanning plane should be parallel or perpendicular to the tendon.

Anatomy

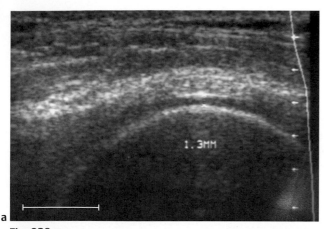 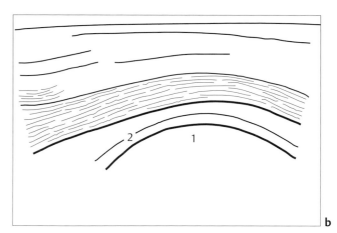

Fig. 328
Posterior longitudinal scan of the medial femoral condyle (**1**), cartilage (**2**) (**a** and **b**).

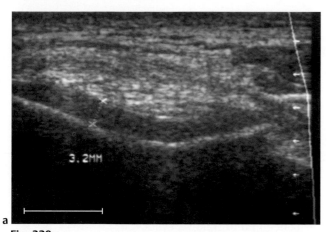 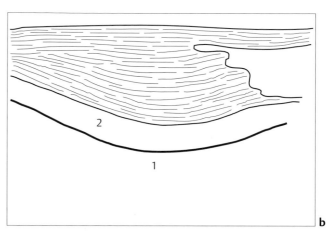

Fig. 329
Anterior transverse scan, knee flexed, trochlea (**1**), trochlear cartilage (**2**) (**a** and **b**).

Ultrasonography may be used to reliably assess both the thickness and the integrity of the articular cartilage of the femoral condyles and intercondylar groove. The knee must be scanned in different degrees of flexion in order to fully visualize the femoral condylar cartilage. The normal cartilage of the femoral condyles and intercondylar groove is a distinct hypoechoic band with sharp anterior and posterior margins. Mean thickness of normal weight-bearing cartilage ranges from 1.2 to 1.9 mm. The patellar articular surface is not accessible by ultrasound.

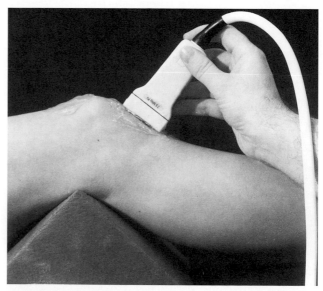

Fig. 330
Position for evaluation of the patellar tendon.

Knee

Effusion

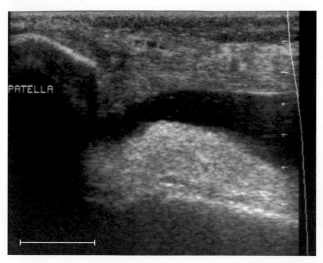

Fig. 331
A fluid-filled suprapatellar pouch is shown in this sagittal scan, lying between the quadriceps tendon and the prefemoral fat.

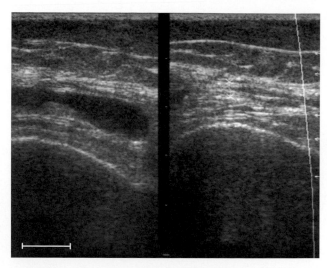

Fig. 332
An axial scan obtained with and without compression of the suprapatellar pouch measures the discrete thickening of the synovial membrane in this patient with rheumatoid arthritis.

Minimal effusions can be detected with ultrasound. They should be looked for not only at the suprapatellar pouch, but also lateral and medial to the patella. The thickness of the anterior and posterior synovial membrane can be measured after compression of the suprapatellar pouch. Comparison with measurements at the contralateral side and evolution of synovial thickness are more important in ascertaining the pathology than absolute values. Loose bodies in primary, or more commonly in secondary osteochondromatosis, should be searched for in the suprapatellar pouch and in Baker's cysts.

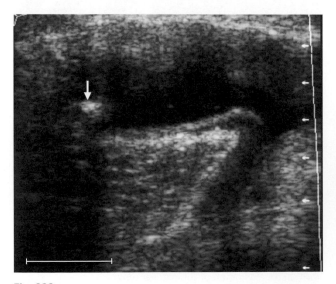

Fig. 333
A hyperechoic loose body (→) is observed in a Baker's cyst.

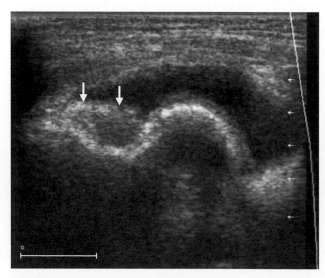

Fig. 334
Fluid surrounding the popliteal tendon (→) is not pathognomonic for tendinitis, but may also be present in joint effusion.

Baker's Cyst

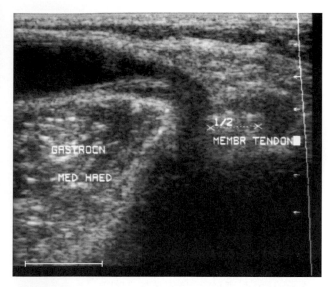

Fig. 335
A Baker's cyst with its base on the medial femoral condyle. The neck corresponds to the semimembranosus-gastrocnemius bursa, the body of the cyst lies over the medial gastrocnemius muscle.

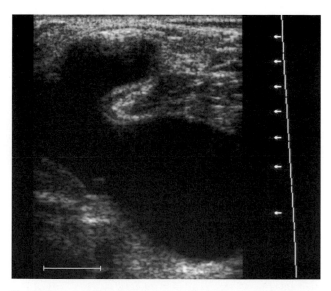

Fig. 336
Superficial and deep extension of a Baker's cyst is observed in a sagittal plane.

Baker's cyst originates in the common semimembranosus-gastrocnemius bursa on the medial femoral condyle. It does not communicate at birth, but communication develops during growth. It can extend distally and superficially, and less frequently deep to the gastrocnemius muscle. Its synovium lined wall becomes thickened with time, or can show synovial proliferation in inflammatory diseases. Loose bodies often accumulate in these cysts. When the normally rounded distal extremity of the cyst becomes tapered, associated with subcutaneous edema and pain resembling thrombophlebitis, the diagnosis of a ruptured Baker's cyst should be suggested. Fascial planes may be dissected by small amounts of fluid originating from the ruptured cyst.

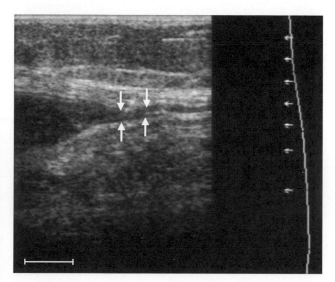

Fig. 337
A tapered extremity (→) of a ruptured Baker's cyst.

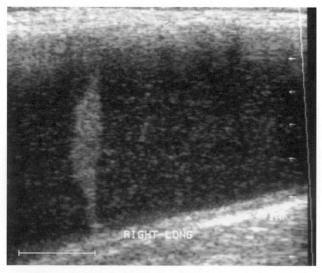

Fig. 338
Echoic contents and synovial proliferation complicated by torsion is responsible for articular pain in this patient with rheumatoid arthritis.

Knee

Popliteal Masses

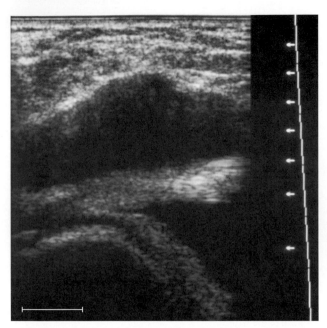

Fig. 339
A typical Baker's cyst, with its medial topography.

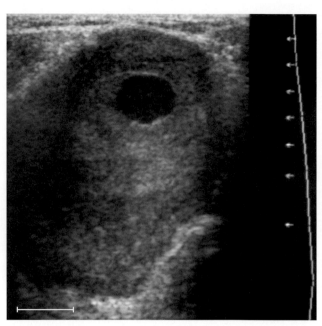

Fig. 340
Popliteal artery aneurysm with large thrombus formation.

Patients are frequently referred for evaluation of a popliteal mass. The most common nonmuscular popliteal masses are Baker's cyst, popliteal aneurysm, venous thrombosis, and neurofibroma. Baker's cysts are anechoic or hypoechoic, located posterior to the medial femoral condyle, and communication with the joint can frequently be observed. Popliteal aneurysms appear as saccular or fusiform widenings of the popliteal artery, with peripheral hypoechoic thrombus and often wall calcifications. In venous thrombosis, the content of the vein is hypoechoic, and the vein is not compressible. Neurofibromas appear as hypoechoic masses along the nerve course.

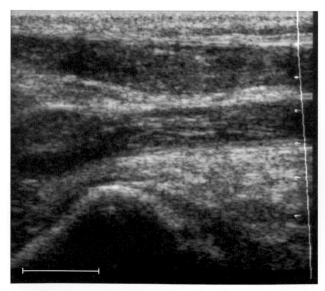

Fig. 341
Deep venous thrombosis of a duplicated popliteal vein.

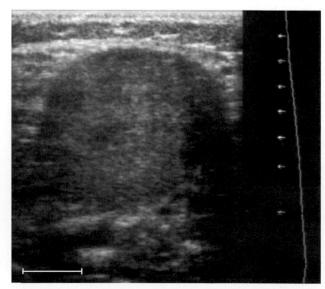

Fig. 342
A neurofibroma in a location posterolateral to the vessels in an axial scan. Bleeding is responsible for the central hyperechogenicity.

Tendinitis

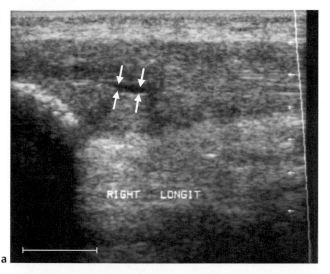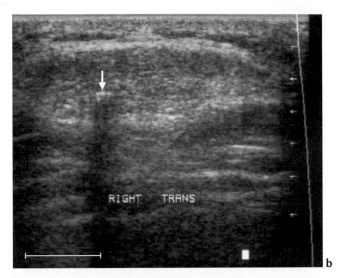

Fig. 343
A hypoechoic thickened proximal patellar tendon (jumper's knee), with a small intrasubstance tear (→) (**a**). A transverse scan of the same patient shows also a small calcification (→) (**b**).

At the knee, tendinitis is frequently observed in the quadricipital, patellar, bicipital, and pes anserinus tendons. Tendinitis is seen as a swelling and hypoechoic appearance of the tendon. Calcifications are rare, but are pathognomonic of a chronic stage. Ultrasound is the only method that can show tendon fibers. In contrast to MRI, ultrasound is able to show microruptures, due to its high resolution. In MRI, a hyperintense signal is seen in tendinitis, as well as in partial rupture.

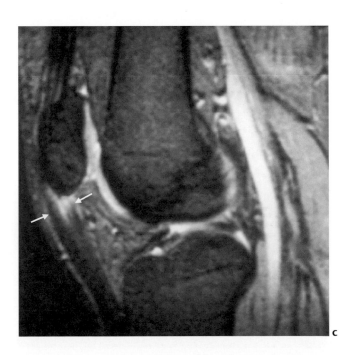

Fig. 343
MRI performed in the same patient shows a hyperintense signal intensity of the thickened patellar tendon at its proximal end (→) (**c**).

Knee

Patellar Tendinitis

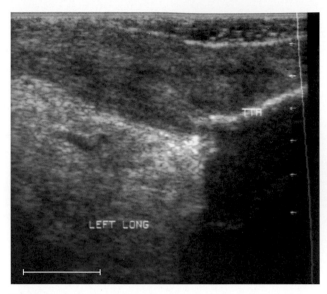

Fig. 344
A diffuse, hypoechoic, thickened patellar tendon with tiny microruptures.

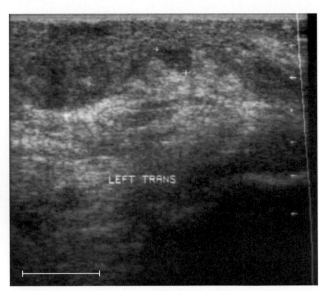

Fig. 345
A transverse scan of a patellar tendinitis shows hypoechoic and hyperechoic nodules. The tendon has indistinct margins.

Acute and chronic tendinitis are not distinct, and a continuous spectrum of ultrasound findings can be seen: diffuse hypoechoic thickening, nodular hypoechoic or hyperechoic thickening, posterior acoustic enhancement, irregular contours of the tendon, and hyperechoic Hoffa's fat. Calcifications are only seen in the chronic stage. Similar changes can also be observed after arthroscopy, when a passage is made through the tendon. Ossification at the entheses is seen in repeated microinjuries, by stimulation of the cartilage at the insertion site of the tendon.

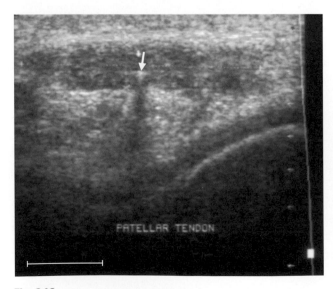

Fig. 346
A calcification (→) reflecting chronic tendinitis in a hypoechoic tendon with nodular formation.

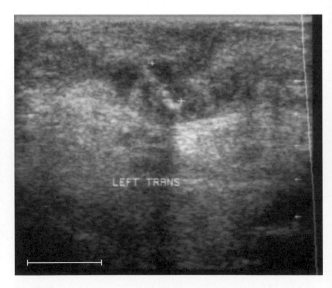

Fig. 347
The linear hypoechoic pathway of a previous arthroscopy. Nodular hypoechoic thickening, diagnostic of tendinitis, is present.

Osgood—Schlatter Disease

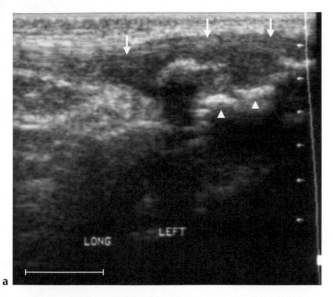
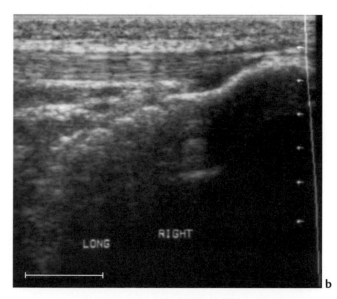

a b

Fig. 348
The patellar tendon has a hypoechoic thickened appearance at its distal end (→). Bone irregularities and a free fragment of the anterior tibial tuberosity are found (▶) (**a**). The distal patellar tendon on the opposite side is normal. The tibial tuberosity has a smooth surface (**b**).

Osgood–Schlatter disease results from repeated microinjuries to the patellar tendon. It is not a true osteochondrosis of the anterior tibial tuberosity. The distal part of the patellar tendon is thickened and hypoechoic, and can contain fragments from the anterior tibial tuberosity. It is often associated with a hyperechoic appearance of Hoffa's fat. There are no specific ultrasound features, compared to tendinitis in general, except for the osseous fragments.

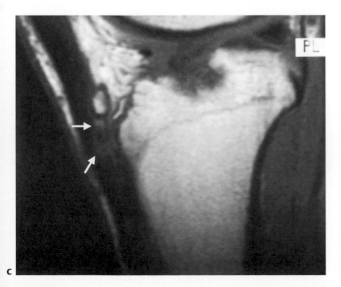
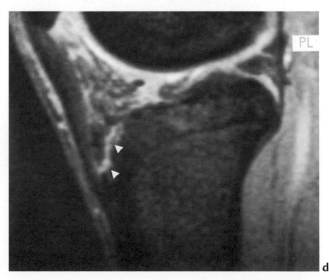

c d

Fig. 348
On MRI, T$_1$-weighted (**c**) and T$_2$-weighted (**d**) images of the same patient show the nonhomogeneous tendon on T$_1$ (→), giving a hyperintense signal on T$_2$ (▶). The fragmented tibial tuberosity is recognized.

Knee

Quadriceps Tendon Rupture and Tendinitis

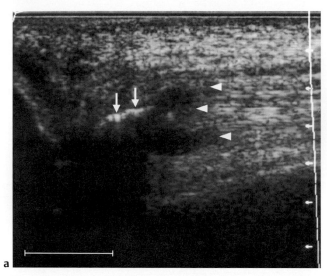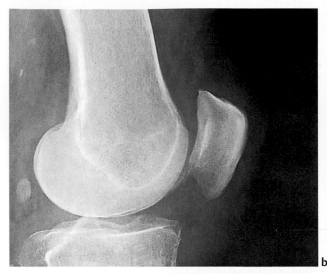

a   b

Fig. 349
An anechoic rupture of the quadriceps tendon (▶) containing an avulsed cortical fragment (→) (**a**). Corresponding plain film (**b**).

Rupture of the quadriceps muscle or tendon occurs with trauma or after excessive muscle contraction. On ultrasound, rupture of the quadriceps tendon is seen as a fluid-filled gap between the patella and the free tendon ends; the extent of the rupture can be measured. Tendinitis is seen as focal hypoechoic indistinct thickening. A calcified enthesopathy is common at the quadriceps tendon insertion.

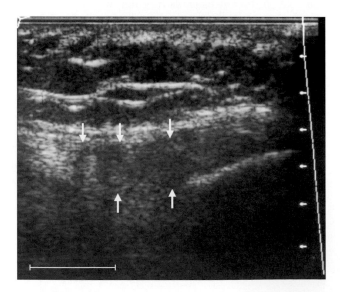

Fig. 350
Heterogeneous hypoechoic focal tendinitis at the insertion of the quadriceps tendon (→).

Pes Anserinus Tendinitis

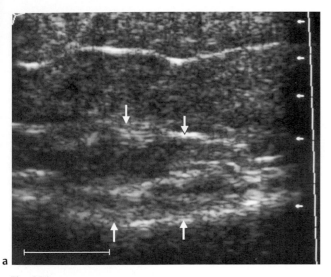 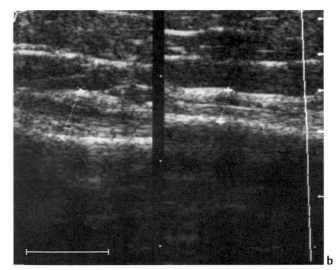

Fig. 351
Tendon thickening (→) separated by a fluid film (**a**). These findings are more obvious in a comparative study (**b**).

The pes anserinus is composed of the tendinous insertions of the sartorius, gracilis, and semitendinosus muscles, inserting in this order from anterior to posterior on the medial tibial metaphysis. A comparative study is mandatory to evaluate the tendon thickness in pes anserinus tendinitis. The tendons are thickened, hypoechoic, and bursitis can be associated.

Retinaculum/ Synovial Impingement

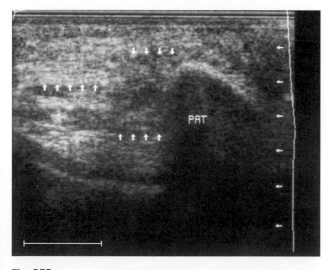 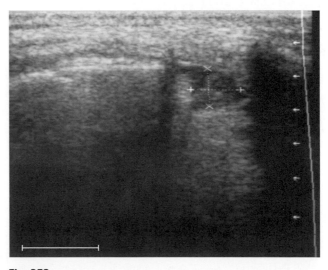

Fig. 352
Interruption of fibers with associated hematoma (→) at the patellar insertion of the medial retinaculum.

Fig. 353
Hypoechoic tender synovial impingement at the outer border of the patella.

Lesions at the medial retinaculum can be found in association with patellar luxation. In acute rupture, the hypoechoic band is interrupted by an anechoic or hypoechoic hematoma. In chronic lesions, the retinaculum remains hyperechoic, but is thickened. A focal synovial impingement between the patella and one of the femoral condyles can have a mechanical origin, such as an osteophyte or a medial synovial plica. Ultrasound shows a tender, hypoechoic nodule.

Knee

Bursitis

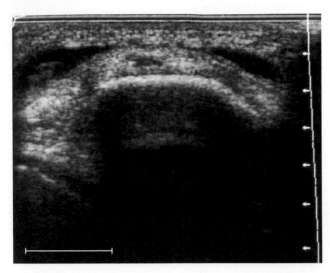

Fig. 354
Prepatellar bursitis due to chronic friction, with anechoic contents and a thickened wall.

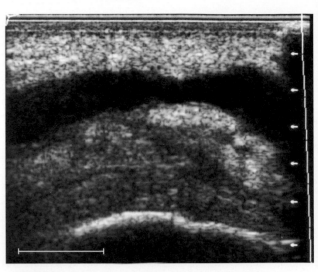

Fig. 355
An acute inflamed prepatellar bursitis is observed in an acute attack of gout. The bursal walls are not yet thickened. Note the diffuse subcutaneous edema, giving a thickened and hyperechoic appearance compared to **Fig. 354**

Prepatellar and deep infrapatellar bursae are non-communicating. They can communicate when a large chronic bursitis is present. Frictional and gouty bursitis are the most frequent pathologies. In frictional bursitis, the content is usually anechoic. Hyperechoic walls and echoic content develop over time. In gouty bursitis, the contents are hypoechoic, sometimes asso-ciated with nodules. In acute forms, the surrounding tissues are edematous. Hemorrhagic bursitis can be observed, especially in patients who participate in contact sports. Hemorrhagic contents are echoic, and may contain echoic blood clots. In case of highly localized prepatellar bursitis, a rupture of the quadricipital tendon has to be ruled out.

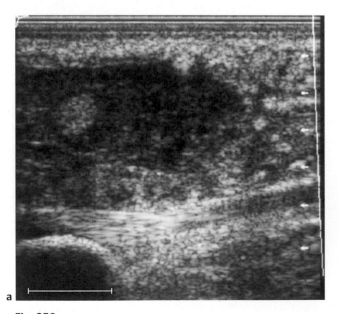

Fig. 356
A large proximal prepatellar bursitis (**a**) communicates with the distal prepatellar bursa in a chronic gouty bursitis with hypoechoic content and hyperechoic nodules. Note also bursitis located deep to the patellar tendon at its distal insertion (→) (**b**).

Medial Collateral Ligament Injury

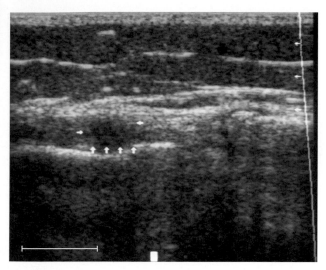

Fig. 357
As a consequence of rupture of the deep layer of the medial collateral ligament, hypoechoic tissue fills the gap (→).

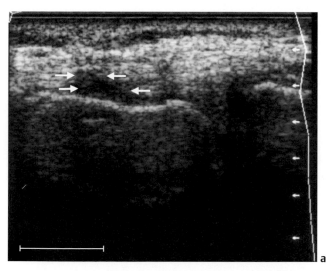

Fig. 358
A rupture of both layers with a hypoechoic gap is shown (→).

Ruptures occur after forceful valgus stress, for instance in soccer players or after arthroscopy. The rupture can be partial, involving the deep layer, or complete. If untreated, a painful granuloma and/or calcification, usually located at the proximal insertion (Stieda–Pellegrini Syndrom) can develop. In sports injuries,

complete rupture of the medial collateral ligament is often associated with anterior cruciate ligament rupture and medial meniscal tear. In acute rupture, one or both hyperechoic bands that form the ligament are separated by hematoma, appearing as an anechoic or hypoechoic cleft. The ligament is thickened.

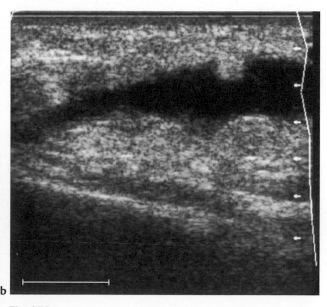

Fig. 358
In the same patient, an anechoic fluid collection dissecting subcutaneous fat has migrated in front of the medial cortex of the proximal tibia.

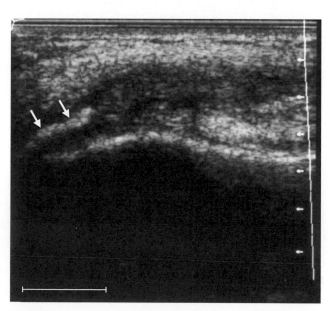

Fig. 359
A hypoechoic nodular granulation tissue is found in this chronic untreated complete rupture, with a calcification (→) at the proximal insertion of the medial collateral ligament (Stieda–Pellegrini's disease).

Knee

Lateral Collateral Ligament Injury

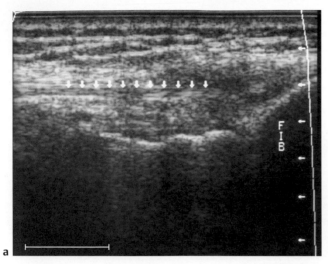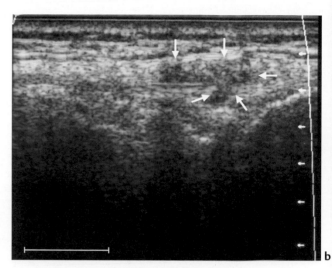

Fig. 360
Two ruptured lateral collateral (→) ligaments and associated hematoma at their distal insertion (**a** and **b**).

The lateral collateral ligament is less frequently injured than the medial one. Lateral meniscal tear and anterior cruciate ligament rupture can be associated lesions. Ultrasound shows the ligamentous discontinuity and the hypoechoic or anechoic hematoma.

Shin Splint

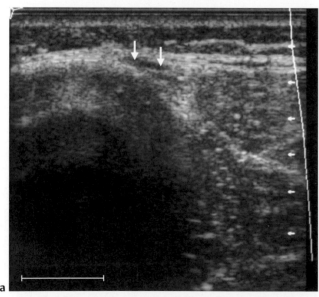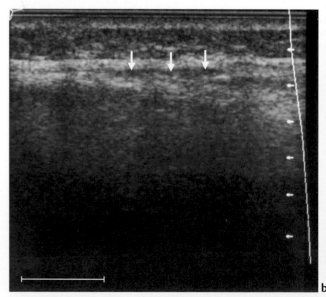

Fig. 361
Thickening and a hypoechoic band in the fascia (→) near the anterolateral tibial cortex in transverse (**a**) and longitudinal (**b**) planes in this trampoline jumper.

A shin splint is a fascial thickening at the anchoring points of the muscular compartments on the lateral or posteromedial border of the tibia. It is related to excessive exercise of the foot flexors. Ultrasound shows fascial thickening and edema. Another traumatic fascial lesion, described as runner's knee, is due to friction of the iliotibial band over the lateral femoral condyle.

Cruciate Ligament Injury

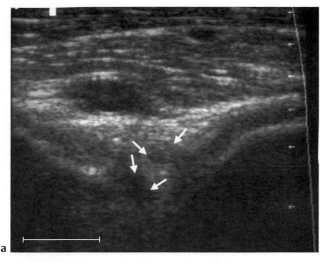 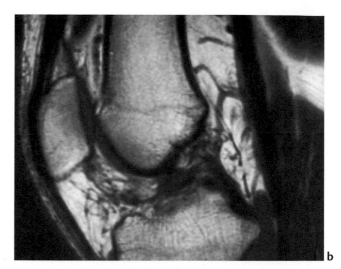

a   b

Fig. 362
An interrupted anterior cruciate ligament (→) in the chronic phase (**a**). Corresponding MRI of the same patient (**b**).

Both cruciate ligaments present as hypoechoic bands, running in an oblique sagittal course (see Figs. **316** and **317**). The anterior cruciate ligament has to be evaluated in full flexion by an anterior approach. This may be impossible in the acute traumatic phase. The posterior cruciate ligament, which is rarely injured, can easily be evaluated by posterior scanning. A partial or complete tear will appear as a mass effect of the ligament, with or without visible interruption.

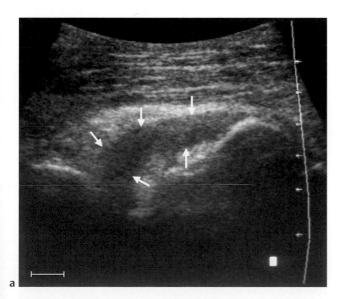 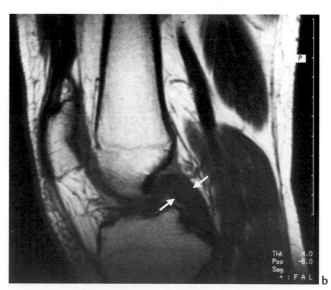

a   b

Fig. 363
A heterogeneous, diffusely swollen aspect of the posterior cruciate ligament after trauma (→) (**a**). The corresponding MRI of the posterior cruciate ligament (→) with intermediate signal intensity and diffuse mass effect suggests a rupture (**b**).

Knee

Meniscal Tear and Cyst

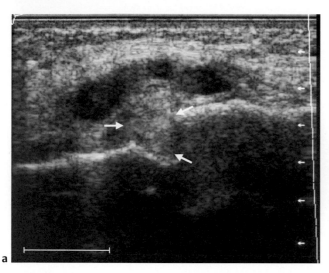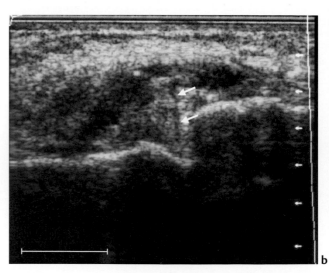

Fig. 364
A fluid collection at the periphery of the internal meniscus (→) separates the intact deep and superficial layers of the medial collateral ligament (**a**). At a different level, the meniscal tear is seen as an anechoic line (→) in the middle of the triangular meniscus (**b**).

Ultrasound is useful in detecting tears, which are peripheral or commmunicate and form meniscal cysts. Most of the meniscus can be evaluated when varus or valgus stress is applied. A meniscal tear appears as a hypoechoic cleft in the meniscus. Ultrasound detects meniscoligamentous separation. Meniscal cysts are associated with tears, and appear as a hypoechoic or hyperechoic mass against the meniscus. They are most frequent on the lateral side. The echogenicity of the cystic content depends on its viscosity. The degenerative meniscus is swollen, hypoechoic, and shows external bulging.

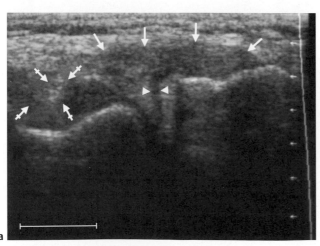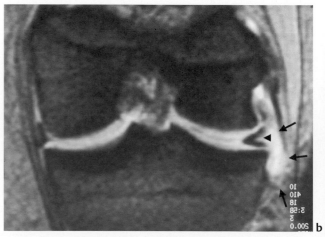

Fig. 365
More echoic content of an external meniscal cyst (→), associated with an anechoic meniscal tear (▶). Note the presence of fluid around the popliteus tendon (↔) in its groove, due to its intra-articular course (**a**). A coronal T$_2$-weighted MRI of the same patient shows the hyperintense meniscal cyst (→) and the tear in the meniscus (▶) (**b**).

Ganglion Cyst

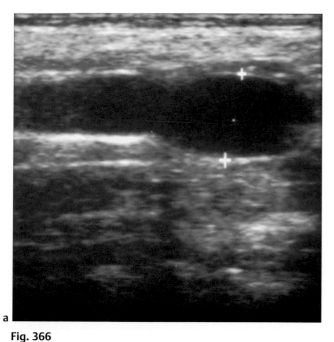
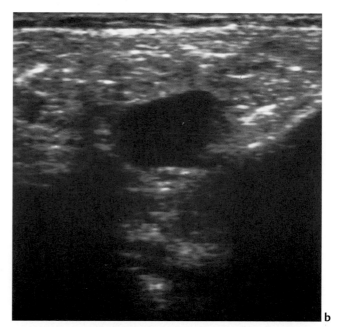

a   b

Fig. 366
This 37-year-old male presented with a step foot. A cystic mass is evident deep to the extensor and tibialis anterior muscle: longitudinal (**a**) and transverse views (**b**).

Ganglion cysts are frequently found at the level of the knee: around or inside the bone, around the cruciate ligaments, in arterial walls, in nerves, and in muscles. Ultrasound can detect these lesions in the soft tissues and demonstrate articular, tendinous, or ligamentous connections. They appear as multiloculate, anechoic or hypoechoic, septated structures. They are not associated with meniscal tears.

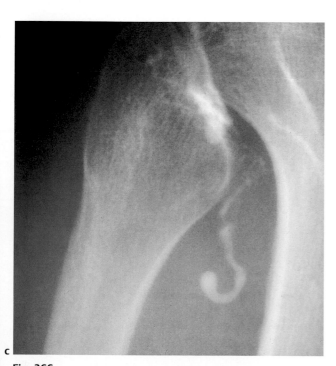
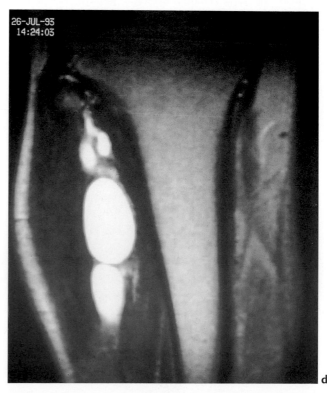

c   d

Fig. 366
Arthrography shows the communication with the proximal tibiofibular joint (**c**). The corresponding T_2-weighted MRI is shown. At surgery, a ganglion cyst was found dissecting the deep peroneal nerve (**d**).

Knee

Periosteal Desmoid

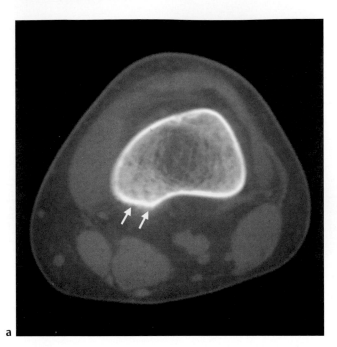

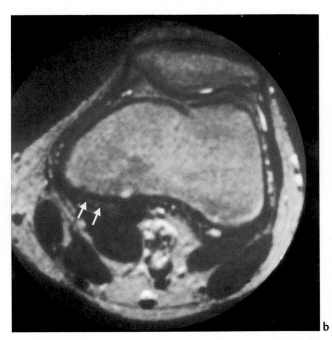

a b

Fig. 367
On CT, a soft–tissue swelling with cortical irregularity and periostitis is noted (→) at the attachment of the medial head of the gastrocnemius muscle (**a**). MRI shows the same lesion (→) and rules out a neoplastic process on a T$_2$-weighted image (**b**).

Cortical periosteal desmoid is a benign lesion of traumatic or microtraumatic origin that can mimic aggressive tumor, even on histologic specimens. It usually occurs on the posteromedial condyle of the femur. Pain is not always experienced. Bone scan can be positive. It occurs in young people, and produces a periosteal reaction on plain films. Ultrasound shows the periosteal reaction as a hyperechoic band displaced from the cortical line. It confirms the absence of tumor in the soft tissues, and localizes the lesion at the insertion site of the medial head of the gastrocnemius muscle.

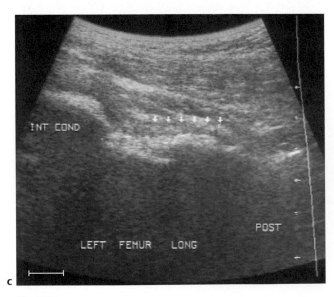

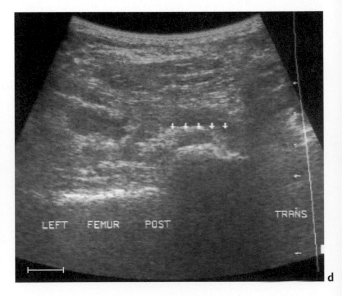

c d

Fig. 367
Ultrasound shows the periosteal reaction as a smooth elevated hyperechoic line (→) at the posteromedial cortex of the distal femur. No mass is seen in the soft tissues (**c** and **d**).

Anatomy

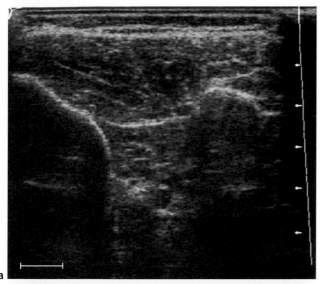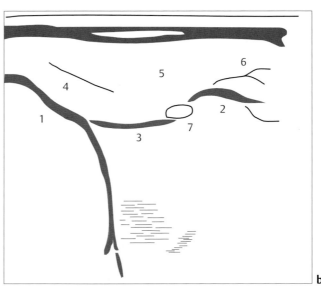

a   b

Fig. 368
Anterolateral transverse scan of the proximal third. Tibia (**1**), fibula (**2**), interosseous membrane (**3**), tibialis anterior (**4**), extensor digitorum (**5**), peroneus longus (**6**) muscles, anterior tibial vessels (**7**) (**a** and **b**).

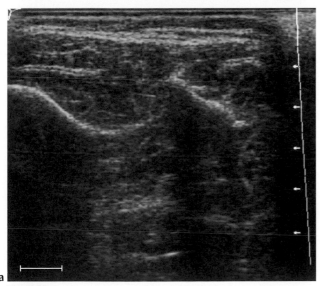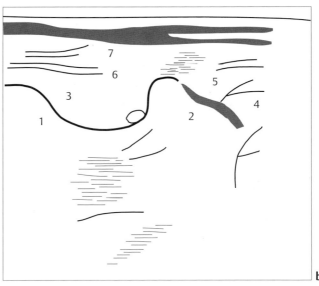

a   b

Fig. 369
Anterior transverse scan of the middle third. Tibia (**1**), fibula (**2**), tibialis anterior (**3**), peroneus longus (**4**), peroneus brevis (**5**), extensor hallucis longus (**6**), extensor digitorum (**7**) muscles (**a** and **b**).

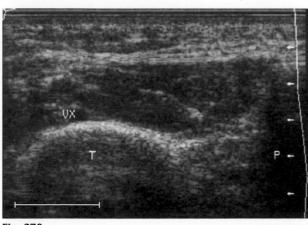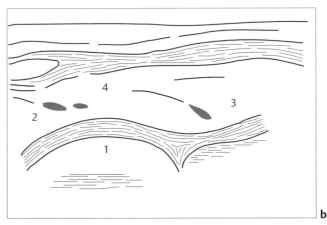

a   b

Fig. 370
Anterior transverse scan of the distal third. Tibia (**1**), tibialis anterior (**2**), extensor digitorum (**3**), extensor hallucis longus (**4**) muscles (**a** and **b**).

Leg

Anatomy

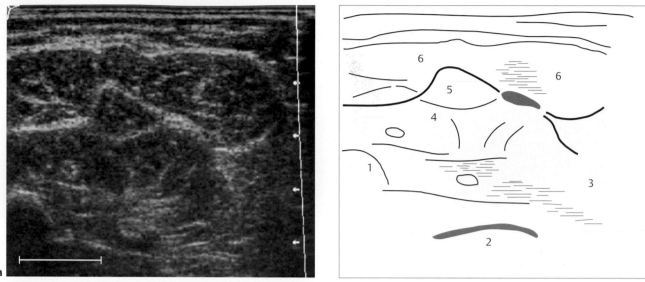

Fig. 371
Posterior transverse scan of the proximal third. Fibula (**1**), tibia (**2**), popliteus (**3**), soleus (**4**), plantaris gracilis (**5**), gastrocnemius (**6**) muscles (**a** and **b**).

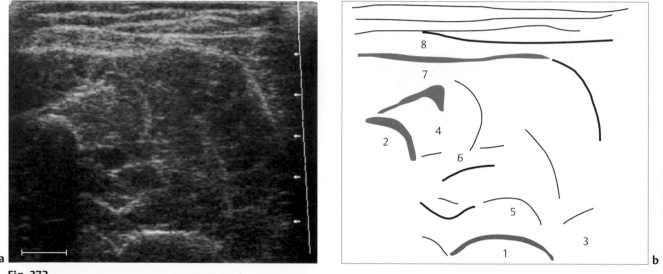

Fig. 372
Posterior transverse scan of the middle third. Tibia (**1**), fibula (**2**), flexor digitorum longus (**3**), flexor hallucis longus (**4**), tibialis posterior (**5**) muscles, posterior tibial vessel (**6**), soleus (**7**), gastrocnemius (**8**) muscles (**a** and **b**).

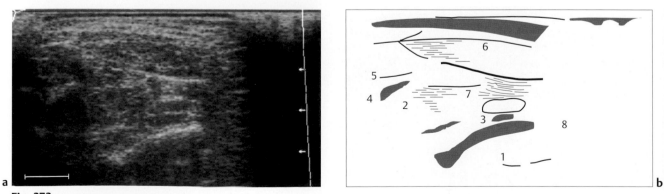

Fig. 373
Posterior transverse scan of the distal third. Tibia (**1**), fibula (**2**), flexor digitorum longus (**3**), peroneus longus (**4**), peroneus brevis (**5**), triceps surae (**6**), flexor hallucis longus (**7**), tibialis posterior (**8**) muscles (**a** and **b**).

Anatomy

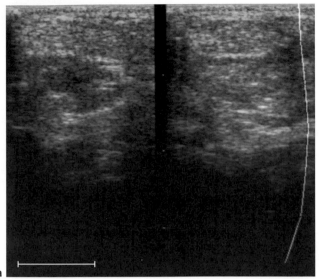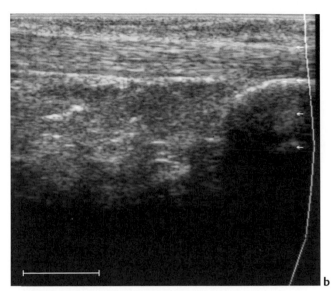

Fig. 374
Transverse scan (**a**) and longitudinal scan (**b**)of the Achilles tendon.

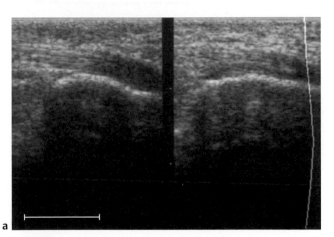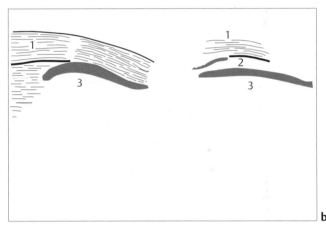

Fig. 375
Longitudinal scans of the Achilles tendon at its insertion (**1**), retrocalcaneal bursa (**2**), calcaneum (**3**) (**a** and **b**).

The Achilles tendon originates from the gastrocnemius and soleus muscles and inserts into the posterior aspect of the calcaneum. The innermost part of the Achilles tendon is formed by the tendon of the plantaris muscle. The muscle fibers at the musculotendinous junction appear linear and hypoechoic, not to be confused with partial tears. The insertion at the posterior calcaneal border also appears hypoechoic due to the oblique course and cartilaginous content of the tendon at this level. The Achilles tendon lies immediately beneath the skin and subcutaneous fat; anterior to the tendon is the less echoic fat of the Kager triangle. The patient is scanned in a prone position; the feet hang over the edge of the table. A dynamic and comparative examination is mandatory. The retrocalcaneal bursa is seen as a fine hypoechoic band interposed between the calcaneum and the tendon.

Ankle

Anatomy

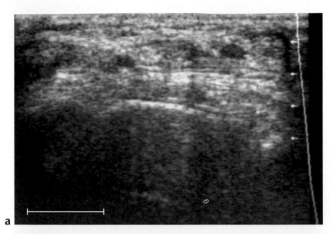
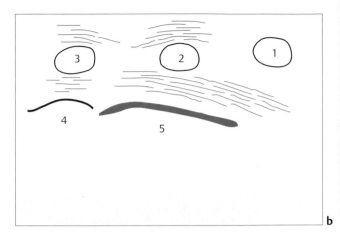

Fig. 376
Anterior transverse scan of the ankle. Tibialis anterior (**1**), extensor hallucis longus (**2**), extensor digitorum longus (**3**) tendons, fibula (**4**), tibia (**5**) (**a** and **b**).

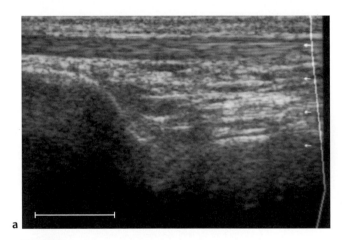
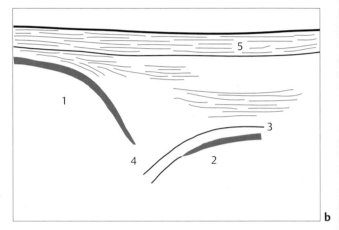

Fig. 377
Anterior longitudinal scan of the ankle. Tibia (**1**), talus (**2**), talar cartilage (**3**), tibiotalar joint (**4**), extensor hallucis longus tendon (**5**) (**a** and **b**).

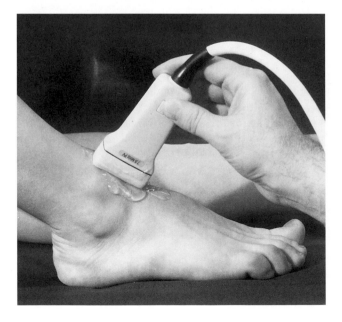

Testing maneuvers are recommended. The Achilles tendon is used as an acoustic window to visualize the posterior articular recess. On an anterior approach, the tibialis anterior tendon is located most medially and has a subcutaneous position anterior to the medial malleolus. The greater saphenous vein is found medial and posterior to it. The extensor hallucis longus tendon lies more lateral, in front of the midportion of the talus. The anterior tibial artery and deep peroneal nerve run posteriorly to this tendon. The extensor digitorum longus is the most lateral tendon, with a small peroneus tendon posteriorly.

Fig. 378
Position for evaluation of the anterior tibiotalar recess and the anterior tendons.

Anatomy

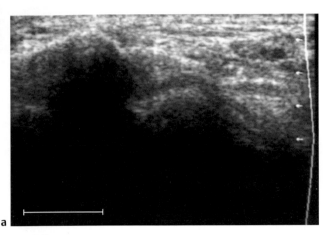
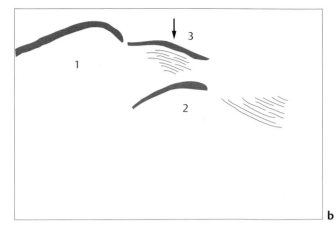

Fig. 379
Transverse scan of the anterior tibiofibular ligament. Fibula (**1**), tibia (**2**), anterior tibiofibular ligament (**3**) (**a** and **b**).

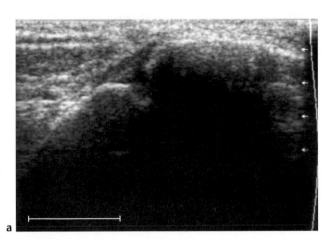
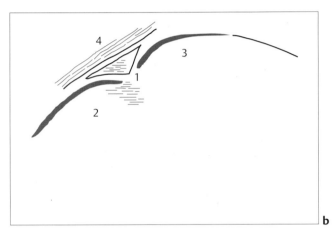

Fig. 380
Transverse scan of the anterior talofibular ligament. Fibulotalar joint (**1**), talus (**2**), fibula (**3**), anterior talofibular ligament (**4**) (**a** and **b**).

The anterior tibiofibular ligament is seen as a hyperechoic band between these two bones. An anterior sagittal scan evaluates the anterior tendons, the anterior tibiotalar recess, and the hyaline cartilage covering the talar dome. The hyperechoic anterior tibiofibular and calcaneofibular ligaments arise from the lateral malleolus. The anterior talofibular ligament runs anteromedially from the anterior margin of the fibular malleolus, forming a tent-like structure over the talus. It attaches to the front of the lateral articular facet and laterally to the neck of the talus and spans the articular space.

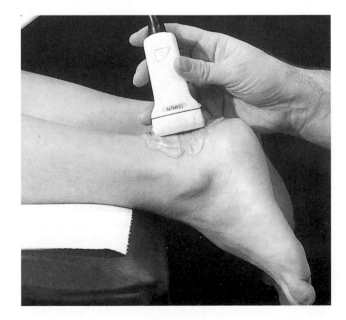

Fig. 381
Position for evaluation of the Achilles tendon and the posterior tibiotalar recess.

Ankle

Anatomy

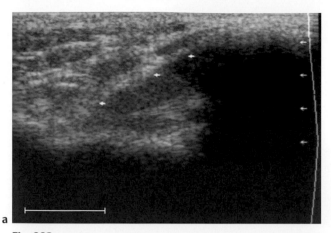
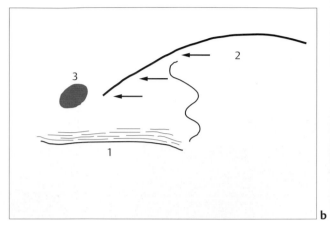

Fig. 382
Longitudinal scan of the lateral malleolus. Calcaneum (**1**), lateral malleolus (**2**), calcaneofibular ligament (→), peroneus tendon (**3**) (**a** and **b**).

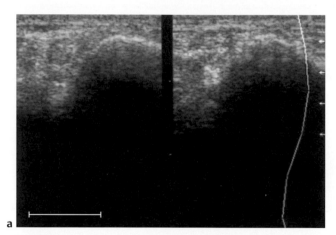
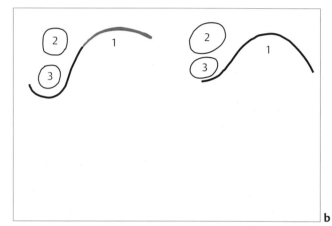

Fig. 383
Transverse scan of the lateral malleolus. Lateral malleolus (**1**), peroneus brevis (**2**), and longus (**3**) tendons (**a** and **b**).

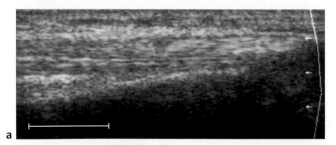
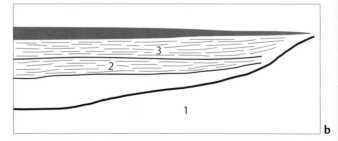

Fig. 384
Longitudinal scan of the lateral malleolus. Lateral malleolus (**1**), peroneus brevis tendon (**2**), peroneus longus tendon (**3**) (**a** and **b**).

The calcaneofibular ligament is examined in a longitudinal plane, slightly dorsal and parallel to the fibular malleolus. The calcaneofibular ligament runs from the apex of the fibular malleolus, caudally and slightly posteriorly to the lateral surface of the calcaneum. This narrow, rounded ligament passes under the tendons of the peroneus longus and brevis muscles. The anterior and posterior tibiotalar ligaments, the tibiocalcaneal and the tibionavicular ligaments arise from the medial malleolus, but are less frequently injured than the other ankle ligaments. The peroneus brevis lies anterior to the peroneus longus tendon in a shallow groove on the posterior aspect of the lateral malleolus. A dynamic examination is obtained in an eversion and dorsiflexion position. The fibers of the peroneus brevis muscle extend distally in the ankle, medial to the corresponding tendon.

Anatomy

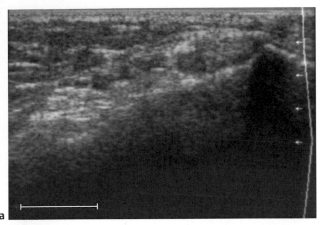
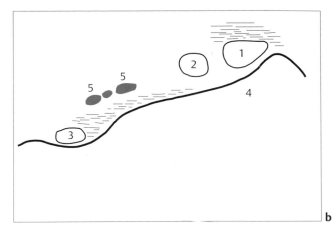

a   b

Fig. 385
Transverse scan at the level of the medial malleolus. Posterior tibialis (**1**), flexor digitorum (**2**), flexor hallucis longus (**3**) tendons, medial malleolus (**4**), posterior tibial vessels and tibial nerve (**5**) (**a** and **b**).

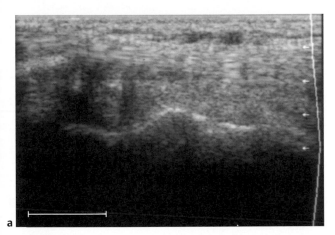
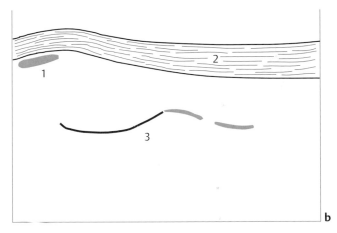

a   b

Fig. 386
Longitudinal scan of the tibialis posterior tendon in its inframalleolar location. Medial malleolus (**1**), tibialis posterior tendon (**2**), talus (**3**) (**a** and **b**).

At the posterior border of the medial malleolus, the tibialis posterior tendon has the most anterior location and is the thickest tendon after the Achilles tendon. The flexor digitorum longus tendon runs immediately posterior to and in close contact with the tibialis posterior tendon. The posterior tibial vessels are found posterior to the flexor digitorum longus tendon accompanied by the tibial nerve. The flexor hallucis longus tendon and muscle occupy an even more posterior tibial position. They lie over the posterior tibial border and are separated from the Achilles tendon by the Kager's triangle.

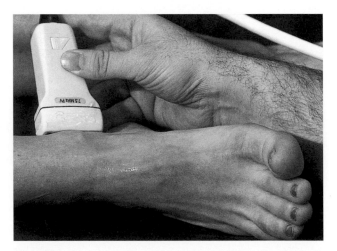

Fig. 387
Position for the evaluation of the tendons behind the medial malleolus.

Ankle

Effusions and Loose Body

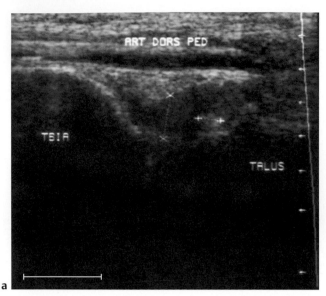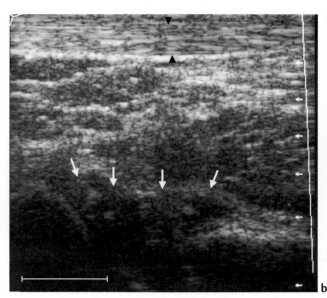

Fig. 388
A distended anterior recess and an intra-articular fragment are shown in a sagittal plane (**a**). A distended posterior recess filled with hyperechoic fragments (→) is observed on a sagittal scan, using the Achilles tendon (▶) as a window (**b**).

Effusions are most obvious at the anterior and posterior tibiotalar recesses, but the lateral and medial joint spaces should also be evaluated. Effusion of various etiologies can be found in association with intra-articular fragments and synovial proliferations, such as in rheumatoid arthritis. Ultrasound is the most appropriate modality for diagnosing loose bodies in the ankle joint.

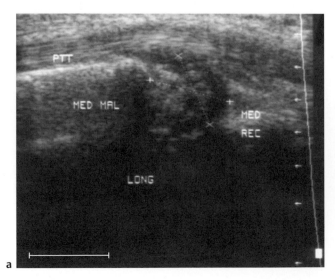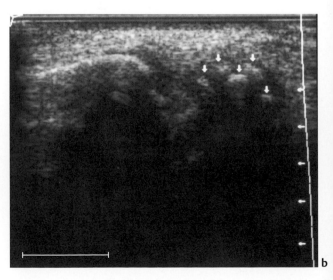

Fig. 389
A capsular distension is seen beneath the medial malleolus, with echoic contents, in this patient with rheumatoid arthritis (**a**). Multiple inframalleolar fragments (→) are found in an external capsular pouch (**b**).

Achilles Tendon Tendinitis

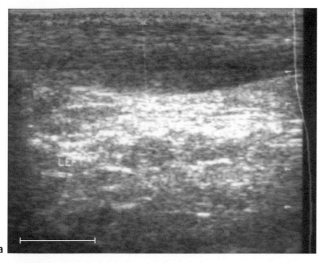
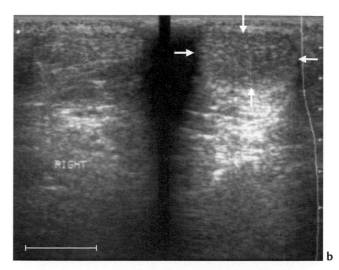

Fig. 390
An acute Achilles tendinitis (→) is shown in a longitudinal scan (**a**). On a transverse scan, a hypoechoic swollen tendon (→) is noted, with posterior acoustic enhancement. Normal opposite side for comparison (**b**).

In acute tendinitis, the Achilles tendon is thickened; it is hypoechoic, but the fibers remain visible. Posterior acoustic enhancement is evident. The anterior border of the tendon is convex on transverse scans. The mar-

gins of the tendon become indistinct, and Kager's fat may be hyperechoic. In chronic tendinitis, calcifications are rarely found, in contrast to patellar tendinitis.

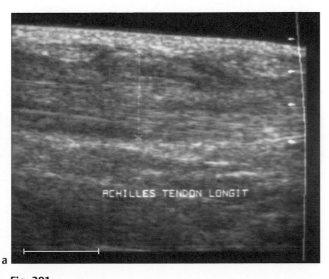
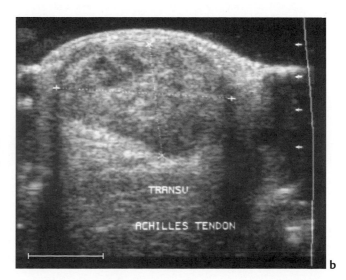

Fig. 391
Longitudinal (**a**) and transverse (**b**) scans of a chronic tendinitis of the Achilles tendon show a swollen, heterogeneous tendon containing nodular formations.

Ankle

Achilles Tendon Tendinitis

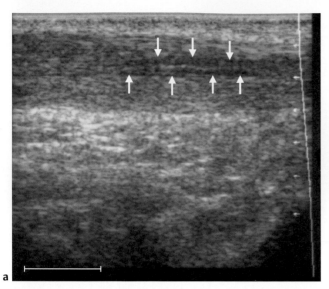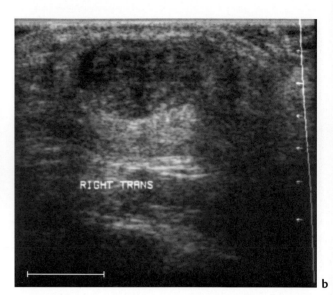

Fig. 392
Longitudinal (**a**) and transverse (**b**) scans of the Achilles tendon reveal acute tendinitis and small, longitudinal fissures (→).

Tendinitis can progress to fissures and partial or complete ruptures. In acute and chronic tendinitis, tiny fissures have to be looked for. Tendinous nodules are sometimes seen on utrasound. Focal tendinitis is rare. A hypoechoic segment of the tendon is more frequently related to partial rupture.

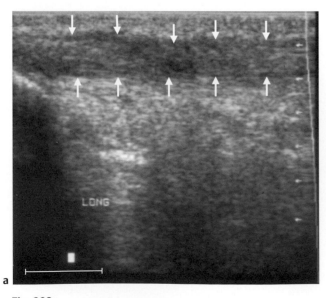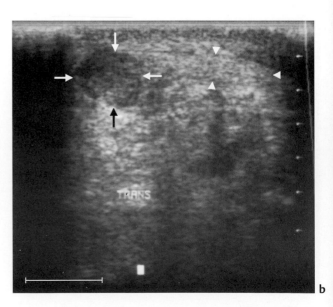

Fig. 393
Tendinitis (→) of the plantaris muscle tendon, located at the medial border of the Achilles tendon (▶), is illustrated in longitudinal (**a**) and transverse (**b**) scans.

Achilles Tendon Rupture

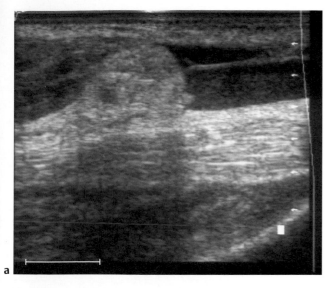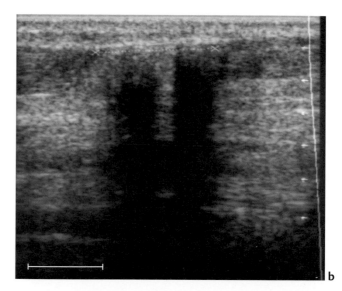

a   b

Fig. 394
A complete tear with a swollen retracted tendon at the musculotendinous junction causes posterior shadowing. Notice the distal anechoic fluid collection (**a**). Complete rupture with refraction at the extremities of the tendon (**b**).

The Achilles tendon is most susceptible to rupture 2–6 cm above the calcaneum. Rupture occurs in athletes, or in previously weakened tendons in patients with rheumatoid arthritis, seronegative spondylarthropathies, systemic lupus erythematosus, gout, or diabetes. Rupture can be missed on clinical examination in 25% of patients. Ultrasound shows an anechoic or heterogeneous hypoechoic defect due to recent hematoma, retracted and swollen ends of the tendon, associated with refraction and shadowing. Fat can fill in the gap. The tendon can have a frayed appearance. In partial rupture, only a part of the tendon has a frayed, hypoechoic appearance, but with a longitudinal extension. The tendon is thickened in its torn part.

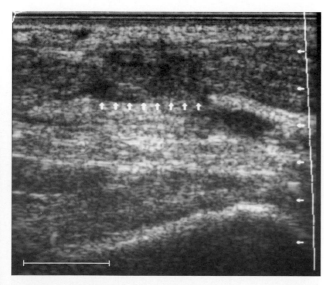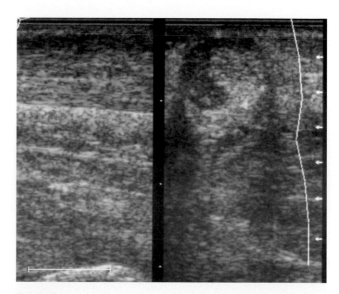

Fig. 395
Complete rupture with a frayed appearance of a hypoechoic Achilles tendon (→).

Fig. 396
Partial rupture with a frayed appearance in longitudinal and transverse planes.

Ankle

Achilles Tendon Rupture

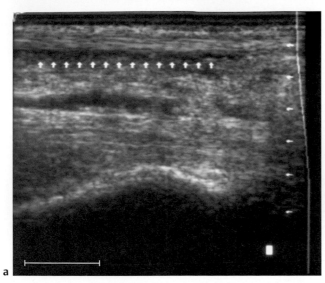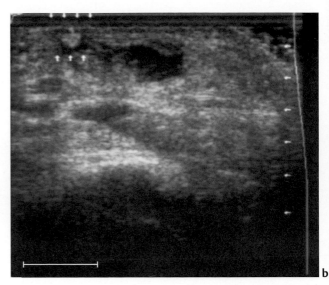

Fig. 397
Longitudinal (**a**) and tranverse (**b**) scans of this complete rupture of the Achilles tendon show an intact tendon of the plantaris muscle
(→).

Conservation of the medial fibers of a ruptured Achilles tendon corresponds to the tendon of the plantaris muscle. If the ends of the ruptured tendon oppose in plantar flexion, conservative treatment can be used.

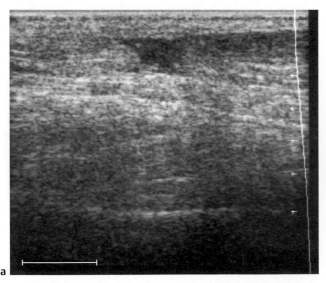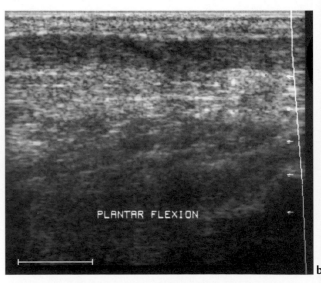

Fig. 398
The ends of the ruptured tendon approach each other in plantar flexion: conservative treatment is advised (**a** and **b**).

Peroneal Tenosynovitis

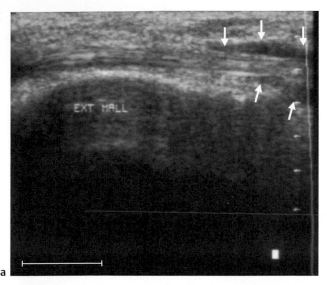 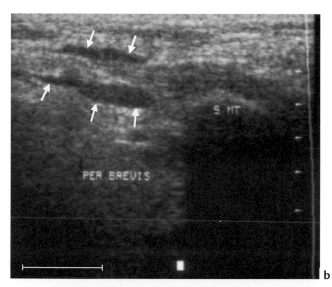

a   b

Fig. 399
Tenosynovitis with a fluid-filled tendon sheath (→) is seen at the retromalleolar level in a coronal plane (**a**). A distended sheath (→) surrounds the peroneus brevis tendon close to its insertion at the base of the fifth metatarsal (**b**).

Tenosynovitis of the peroneal tendons is seen in ankle sprain, in tendinitis or tendon rupture, or in inflammatory conditions. After injury, the fluid is often anechoic. In chronic or inflammatory diseases, the synovial sheath can be thickened, and/or the contents can be more echoic. Peroneal tendon injury is one of the major complications of intra-articular calcaneal fractures. Rupture of the peroneal tendon may cause chronic ankle instability.

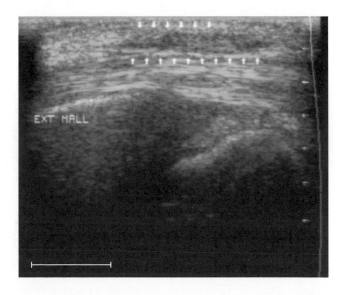

Fig. 400
Synovial thickening of the tendon sheath (→) is observed at the tip of the lateral malleolus in chronic tenosynovitis in this patient with rheumatoid arthritis.

Peroneal Tendon Luxation

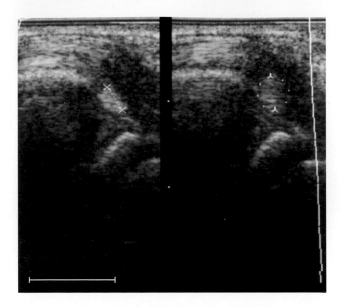

Fig. 401
A mild form of subluxation at the malleolar tip in a coronal scan. The peroneus brevis tendon is displaced anteriorly on dorsiflexion and eversion.

Anterior luxation or subluxation of the peroneal tendons out of their groove in the distal fibula can be caused by loosened or ruptured superior peroneal retinaculum or a dysplastic peroneal tendon groove. A frequent cause of rupture is skiing injuries. Clinically, the patient experiences pain and hears a snap or click.

The luxation or subluxation is tested by dorsiflexion and eversion. Ultrasound will show the displacement of the tendons during dynamic tests. Other secondary signs later in the disease are tenosynovitis, tendon thickening, or rupture.

Peroneal Tendon Rupture

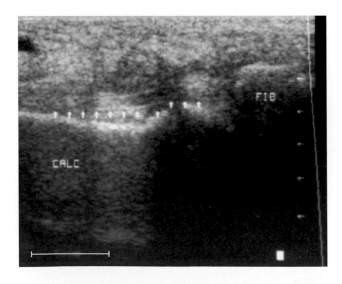

Fig. 402
Rupture of the peroneus longus tendon (→) is seen in its inframalleolar portion.

Peroneal tendon rupture can be partial or complete, longitudinal or transverse. Anechoic or hypoechoic clefts are observed in the tendon, and the amount of fluid in the synovial sheath is usually increased. A dysplastic peroneal tendon groove can be a predisposing factor to fissures.

Posterior Tibial Tendon Tenosynovitis

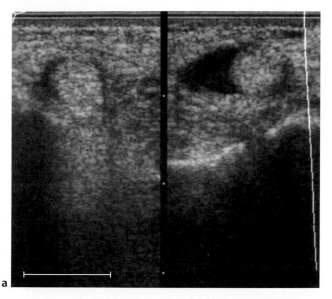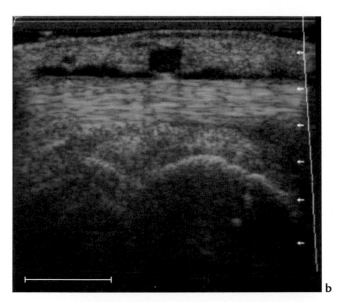

Fig. 403
Tenosynovitis of the posterior tibial tendon is seen in a transverse plane behind the medial malleolus. Tendon thickening and effusion in the tendon sheath is observed (**a**). Effusion and thickening are also seen in an oblique coronal plane along the tendon (**b**).

Evaluation of the posterior tibial tendon is best performed on transverse scans, because on longitudinal views, the pressure of the transducer shifts away the fluid surrounding the tendon. In tenosynovitis, the tendon is surrounded by hypoechoic or anechoic fluid giving a target image on transverse scans. A tendinitis or an associated partial rupture has to be looked for.

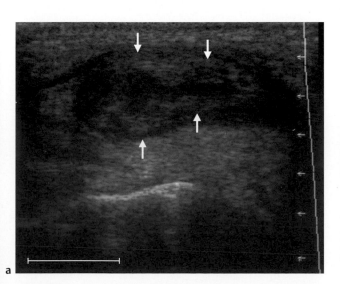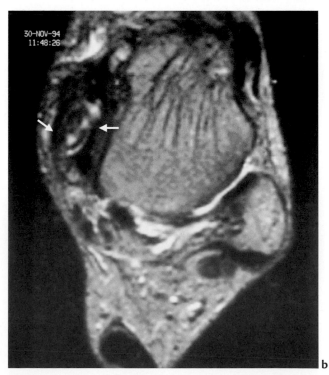

Fig. 404
This patient with long-standing untreated tenosynovitis shows a longitudinal fissure of the thickened inframalleolar part of the tendon (→), better seen with ultrasound (**a**) than on MRI (→) (**b**).

Ankle

Posterior Tibial Tendon Rupture

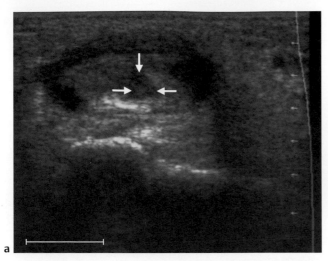 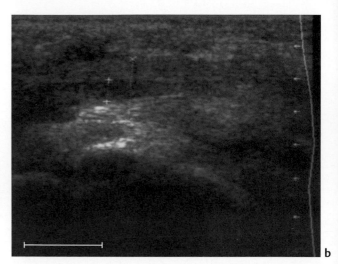

Fig. 405
In this 50-year-old female with a painful flat foot, a longitudinal fissure (→), cleaving the posterior tibial tendon in its inframalleolar portion, is seen in a tranverse scan (**a**). In the longitudinal scan, the gap is 2.8mm and the total tendon thickness 8 mm (**b**).

Rupture of the posterior tibial tendon can cause a flat foot in adults. Normally, this tendon inverts the hindfoot, so that the midtarsal joint becomes rigid and allows the gastrocnemius-soleus muscle to transmit plantar flexion forces to the metatarsal heads. If the posterior tibial tendon is torn, the action of the antagonist peroneus brevis tendon is unopposed, and results in planovalgus deformity. On ultrasound, there is loss of architecture of the tendon fibers. The tendon is interrupted by fluid or echoic material, and tenosynovitis is often associated. Transverse ruptures are most frequently seen underneath the medial malleolus or at the distal insertion. Longitudinal fissures are also seen.

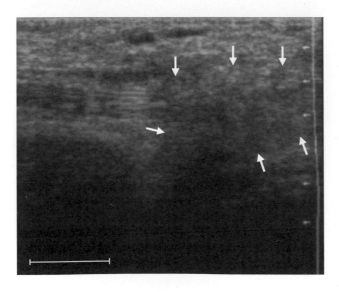

Fig. 406
Chronic rupture of the tendon at its insertion (→), with echoic granulation tissue replacing the tendon.

Bursitis

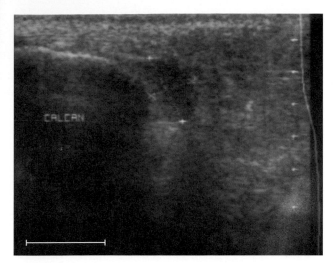

Fig. 407
Retrocalcaneal bursitis is found, in addition to a swollen hypoechoic tendon, in this patient with known ankylosing spondylitis.

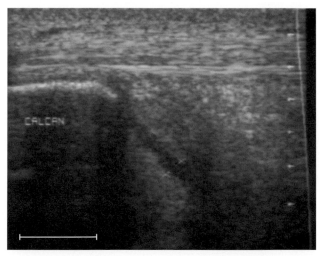

Fig. 408
A small retrocalcaneal bursitis with a thick wall reflecting chronicity and a normal appearing Achilles tendon.

Retrocalcaneal bursitis can be present with or without an associated Achilles tendon tendinitis. The bursitis appears as an anechoic or hypoechoic pouch, located between the anterior aspect of the Achilles tendon and the postero-superior border of the calcaneum. This bursa is enlarged in inflammatory diseases, such as rheumatoid arthritis or seronegative spondylarthropathies, or in frictional bursitis. De novo bursa formation can also be found around the ankle.

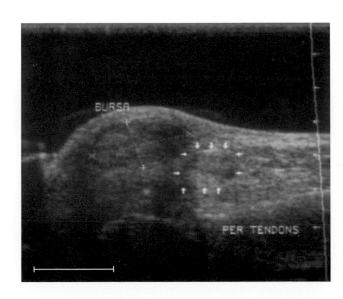

Fig. 409
A de novo bursa formation in contact with the anterior border of the calcaneum underneath the peroneal tendons (→), seen in a coronal plane.

Ankle

Ligament Injury

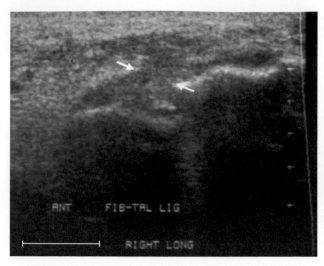

Fig. 410
A tear (→) in the anterior talofibular ligament appears as a gap filled with hypoechoic granulation tissue after one week of immobilization.

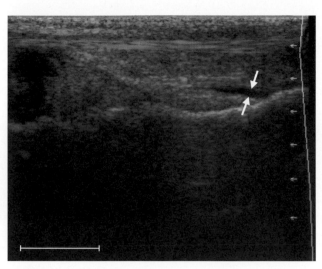

Fig. 411
A partial tear (→) in the deltoid ligament is seen as an anechoic fluid collection at the talar end.

Ultrasound can reveal ligamentous lesions as complete or partial tears, or can show painful nodular granulation tissue after inadequate or absent treatment. Ultrasound is useful in acute sprains, when dynamic studies on plain films are impossible to obtain. Ultrasound is more appropriate than MRI because of the complex orientations of these ligaments. The anterior talofibular ligament runs anteriorly and slightly in-feriorly from the anterior aspect of the distal fibula to the lateral aspect of the talus. The posterior talofibular ligament is short and horizontal. The calcaneofibular ligament is directed slightly posteriorly. In 70% of ankle sprains, only the anterior talofibular ligament is torn. The calcaneofibular ligament is also torn in 20% of cases.

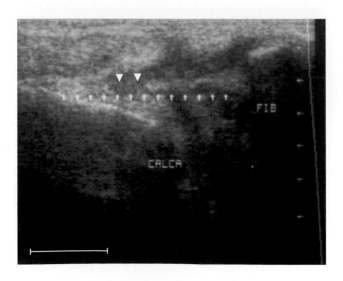

Fig. 412
A complete tear (▶) of the calcaneofibular ligament (→) with its proximal end surrounded by hematoma.

Accessory Soleus Muscle

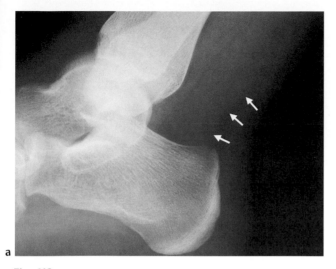
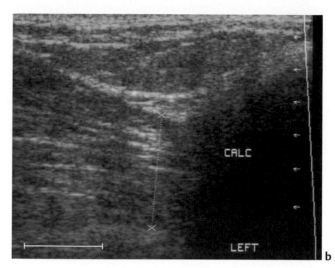

Fig. 413
This 14-year-old ballet dancer complained of a tender posterior mass in the right ankle. The plain film (**a**) shows an opacity with fluid density (→) occupying Kager's triangle. Ultrasound confirms an accessory soleus muscle inserting on the superior calcaneal border (**b**).

The accessory soleus muscle is an unusual anatomical variant in the ankle region. It presents as a mass on the posteromedial aspect of the ankle, and arises from the anterior surface of the soleus muscle or from the fibula and the soleal line of the tibia. Its distal insertion lies on the Achilles tendon or on the medial or superior border of the calcaneum. Clinical symptoms due to an accessory soleus muscle include swelling and pain in the posteromedial aspect of the ankle. This accessory muscle has a poor blood supply, and it is therefore more susceptible to rupture.

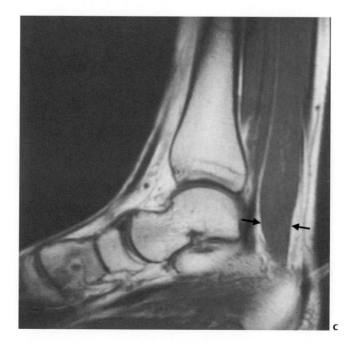

Fig. 413
This accessory soleus muscle (→) is also demonstrated on a T$_1$-weighted MRI in a sagittal plane (**c**).

Ankle

Haglund Deformity

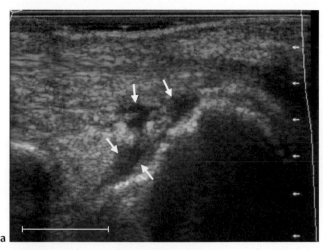
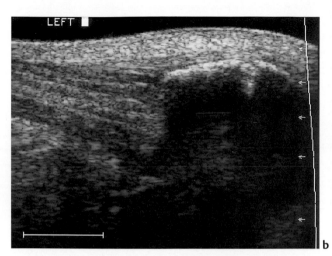

Fig. 414
Retrocalcaneal bursitis (→) and focal skin thickening are seen in this clinically evident Haglund deformity (**a**). Note the thickening of the skin and Achilles tendon (**b**).

Haglund deformity corresponds to a painful posterior bump at the level of the superior calcaneal margin, due to excessive compression of the Achilles tendon. It is associated with a particular morphology of the calcaneum: the angle between the inferior and the posterior border is more than 70°. Ultrasound can reveal focal thickening of the skin, the subcutaneous tissue, and the Achilles tendon in front of the posterior and superior aspect of the calcaneum. Sometimes a small de novo bursa is found in the subcutaneous tissue. Retrocalcaneal bursitis and tendon calcifications are other possible findings, but calcified enthesophytes can also be related to other conditions, such as diffuse idiopathic skeletal hyperostosis (DISH).

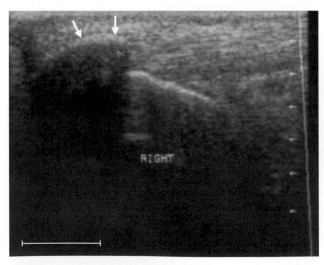
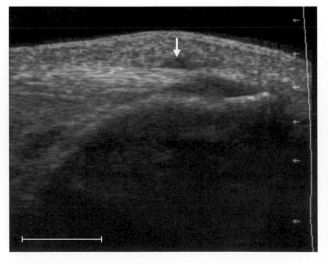

Fig. 415
Calcified insertion enthesopathy (→).

Fig. 416
Focal thickening of retrocalcaneal subcutaneous tissue is associated with de novo bursitis (→).

Cystic Masses

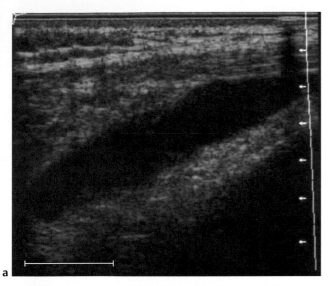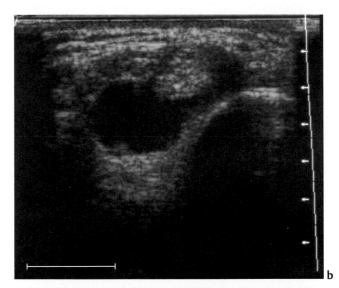

Fig. 417
A tenosynovial cyst arising from the posterior tibial tendon in a superoposterior direction (**a**). A transverse scan shows the base of the cyst (**b**).

Ganglion cysts are frequently described at the level of the ankle joint. They appear as simple, or more often multiloculated, masses with an anechoic or hypoechoic content. They have no true synovial lining, and communication with the joint is rarely found. Other causes of cystic masses are bursitis adjacent to the Achilles tendon, de novo bursitis, and tenosynovial cysts, which appear as anechoic masses arising from a tendon sheath.

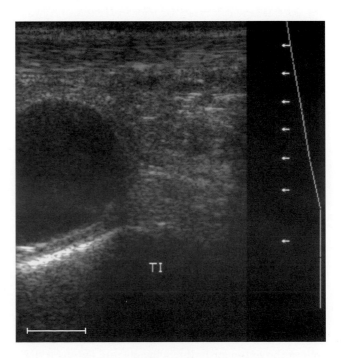

Fig. 418
A cystic mass is found in Kager's triangle posterior to the Achilles tendon and anterior to the posterior tibial cortex. No effusion is noted in the ankle joint. At surgery, a ganglion cyst was resected.

Foot

Anatomy

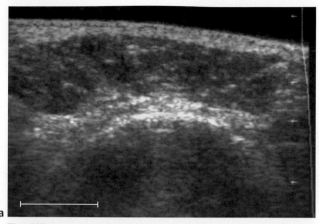
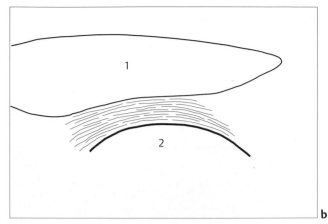

Fig. 419
Laterodorsal coronal scan at the level of the cuboid bone. Extensor digitorum brevis muscle (**1**), cuboid bone (**2**) (**a** and **b**).

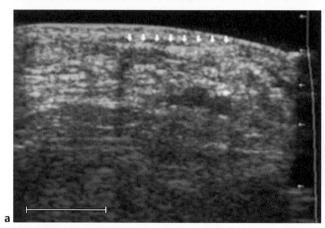
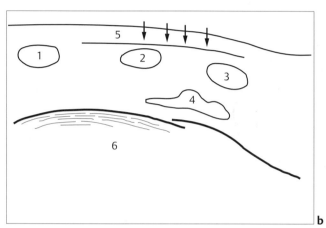

Fig. 420
Mediodorsal coronal scan of the talus. Tibialis anterior (**1**), extensor hallucis longus (**2**), extensor digitorum longus (**3**) tendons, vessels (**4**), annular ligament (→) (**5**), talus (**6**) (**a** and **b**).

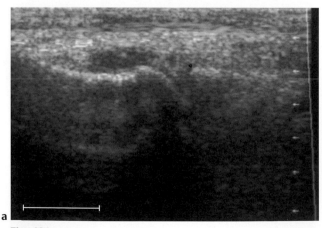
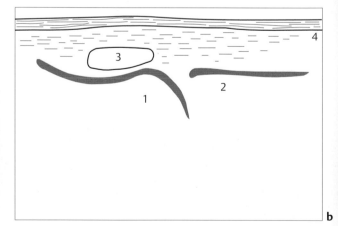

Fig. 421
Sagittal scan of the dorsal aspect of the first metatarsophalangeal joint. First metatarsal (**1**), first phalanx (**2**), extensor hallucis brevis muscle (**3**), extensor hallucis longus tendon (**4**) (**a** and **b**).

From medial to lateral, the tibialis anterior tendon, the extensor hallucis longus tendon, and extensor digitorum longus tendon are seen in the dorsal aspect of the midfoot. The extensor digitorum longus tendon covers the extensor hallucis brevis and extensor digitorum brevis muscles at the level of the cuneiform bones. The hyaline cartilage, the hypoechoic synovial membrane, and the hyperechoic joint capsule can be evaluated as in other synovial joints.

Anatomy

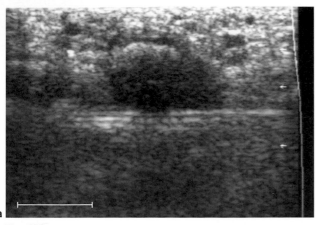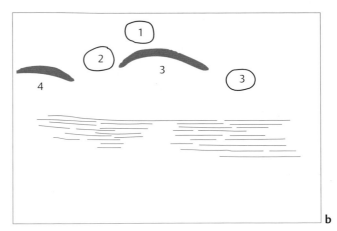

Fig. 422
Dorsal coronal scan at the level of the metatarsal head. Extensor digitorum longus tendon (**1**), dorsal interosseus muscle (**2**), second metatarsal head (**3**), third metatarsal head (**4**) (**a** and **b**).

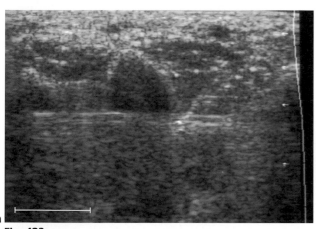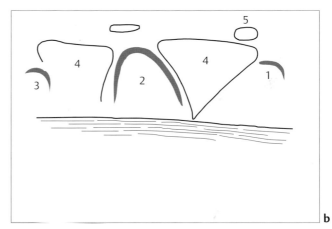

Fig. 423
Dorsal coronal scan at the level of the metatarsal diaphysis. First (**1**), second (**2**), third metatarsal (**3**), dorsal interosseus muscle (**4**), vessels (**5**) (**a** and **b**).

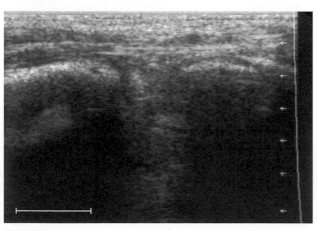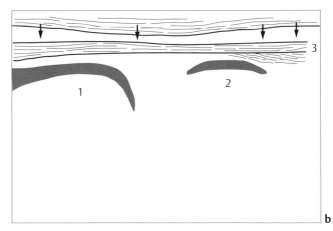

Fig. 424
Transverse scan at the level of the peroneus brevis tendon insertion (**3**), cuneiform (**1**), fifth metatarsal (**2**) (**a** and **b**).

On a transverse scan, the peroneus tendons can be evaluated in their inframalleolar course; the peroneus brevis tendon is in the most anterior position and attaches to the base of the fifth metatarsal. The peroneus longus tendon turns under the inferior border of the calcaneum and cuboid bone and continues in a transverse plantar course.

Foot

Anatomy

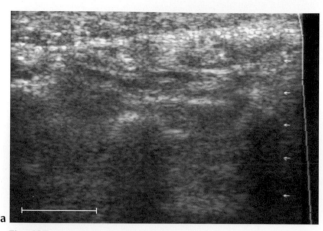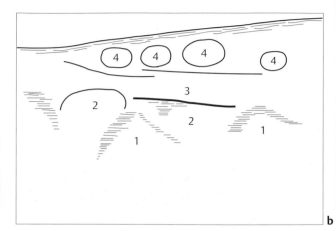

Fig. 425
Plantar coronal scan at the level of the metatarsal bone diaphysis. Metatarsal bone (**1**), interosseous muscle (**2**), flexor digitorum longus (**3**), flexor digitorum brevis tendons (**4**) (**a** and **b**).

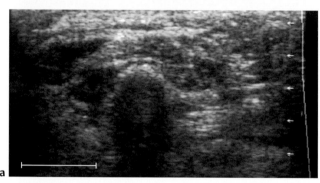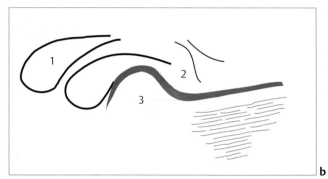

Fig. 426
Lateroplantar coronal scan at the level of the metatarsal bone. Abductor digiti minimi (**1**), flexor digiti minimi muscle (**2**), fifth metatarsal (**3**) (**a** and **b**).

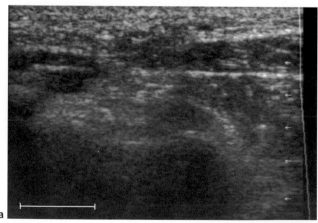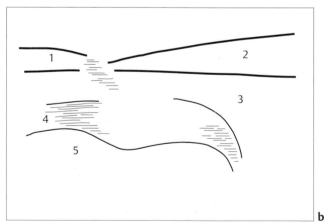

Fig. 427
Lateroplantar coronal scan at the level of the calcaneum. Abductor digiti minimi (**1**), flexor digitorum brevis (**2**), quadratus plantaris (**3**), peroneus longus muscle (**4**), calcaneum (**5**) (**a** and **b**).

The tibialis posterior tendon is oriented horizontally in its inframalleolar course and inserts on the navicular bone. This tendon is in contact with the tibiocalcaneal and spring ligaments, which are located deeper. The flexor digitorum tendon has a more vertical course below the medial malleolus and along the inferior surface of the sustentaculum tali, accompanied by the flexor hallucis longus tendon.

Anatomy

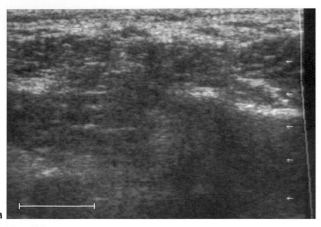
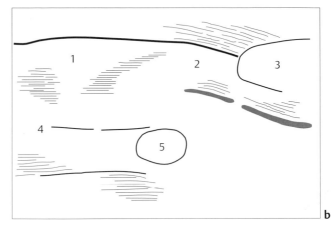

a · b

Fig. 428
Medioplantar coronal scan at the level of the cuneiforms. Flexor digitorum brevis (**1**), flexor hallucis brevis (**2**), abductor hallucis longus (**3**), quadratus plantaris (**4**) muscles, flexor digitorum longus tendon (**5**) (**a** and **b**).

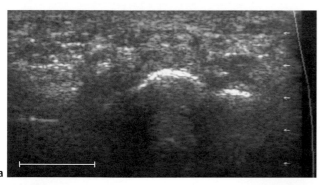
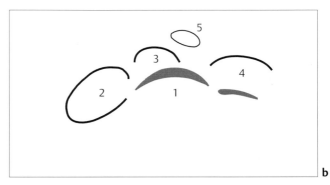

a · b

Fig. 429
Medioplantar coronal scan at the level of the first metatarsal bone. First metatarsal (**1**), abductor hallucis (**2**), flexor hallucis brevis (**3**) muscles, adductor hallucis muscle and tendon (**4**), flexor hallucis longus tendon (**5**) (**a** and **b**).

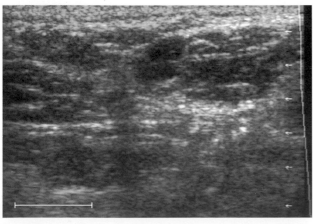
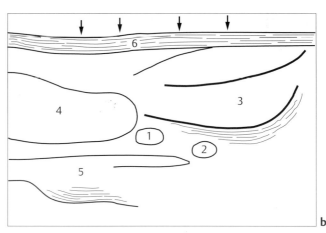

a · b

Fig. 430
Medioplantar transverse scan at the level of the calcaneum. Flexor hallucis longus (**1**), flexor digitorum longus tendon (**2**), adductor hallucis (**3**), flexor digitorum brevis (**4**), quadratus plantae (**5**) muscles, plantar aponeurosis (→) (**6**) (**a** and **b**).

In the plantar aspect of the foot, the adductor hallucis muscle can be found medially, the flexor digitorum brevis muscle centrally, and the abductor digiti minimi laterally. The quadratus plantaris muscle lies deep to the flexor digitorum brevis muscle; the vascular and neural structures lie in between. More distally, the small abductor digiti minimi and adductor hallucis muscles are seen at the inferolateral border of the base of the fifth and first metatarsal. The interosseus muscles are found distally in the intermetatarsal spaces; the flexor digitorum tendons have a more superficial plantar location.

Foot

Anatomy

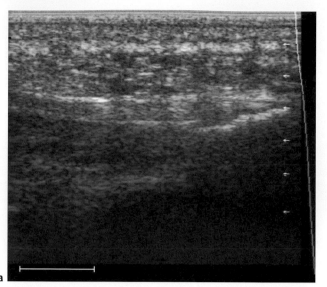
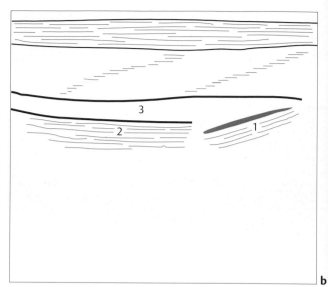

Fig. 431
Midsagittal plantar scan at the level of the calcaneum. Calcaneum (**1**), flexor digitorum brevis muscle (**2**), plantar aponeurosis (**3**) (**a** and **b**).

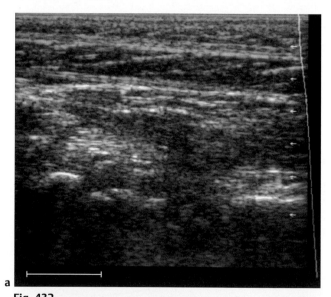
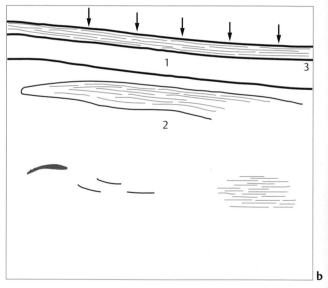

Fig. 432
Midsagittal plantaris scan of the middle of the foot. Flexor digitorum brevis (**1**), quadratus plantaris muscle (**2**), plantar aponeurosis (→) (**3**) (**a** and **b**).

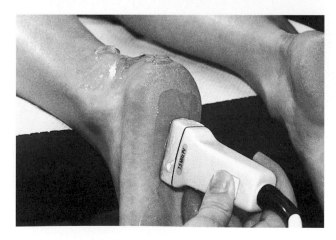

The hyperechoic plantar aponeurosis covers the plantar aspect of the flexor digitorum brevis muscle and has a lateral cord covering the proximal half of the abductor digiti minimi muscle. A midsagittal scan shows the hyperechoic plantar fascia attached to the calcaneum and flexor digitorum brevis. Measurements of the thickness of the plantar sole can be obtained on a transverse scan of the posterior plantar region.

Fig. 433
Position for the evaluation of the plantar fascia.

Rheumatoid Arthritis

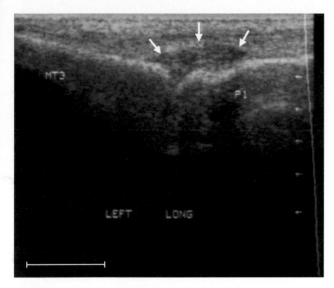

Fig. 434
Synovial capsular thickening (→) at the metatarsophalangeal joint of the third toe, seen in a longitudinal scan.

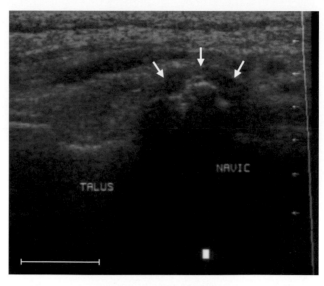

Fig. 435
Synovial proliferations and bone irregularities (→) at the talonavicular joint.

In rheumatoid arthritis of the foot, ultrasound can detect joint effusions and synovial proliferation in the joints and tendon sheaths. Joint effusions with a hypoechoic content are seen more frequently at the metatarsophalangeal joint, and are classically bilateral.

The synovial lining is thickened. Bone erosions can be seen, especially on the lateral aspect of the fifth metatarsal head, sometimes associated with a hypoechoic nodule that forms the pannus. Tarsal joints may be involved.

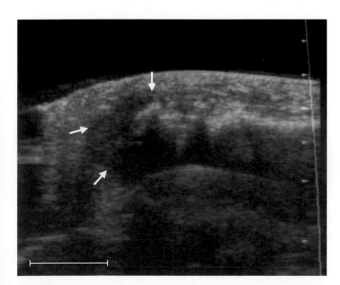

Fig. 436
Hypoechoic pannus formation and erosions at the fifth metatarsophalangeal joint.

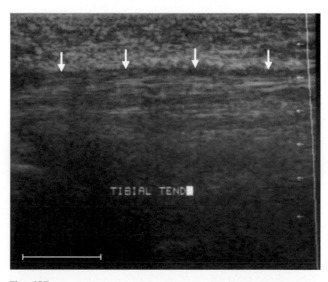

Fig. 437
Synovial thickening (→) of the sheath of the anterior tibial tendon.

Foot

Gout

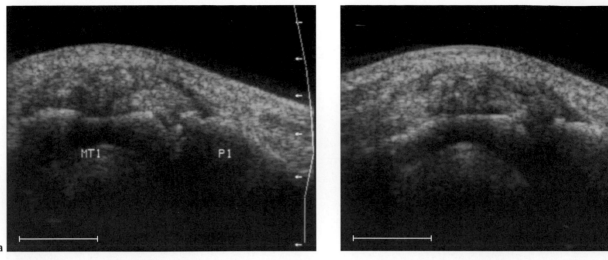

Fig. 438
Soft-tissue swelling with hyperechoic nodules medial to the metatarsophalangeal joint, causing superficial bone erosions (**a** and **b**).

In gout, hypoechoic nodules that may contain calcifications are observed over the medial aspect of the first metatarsal head, which is a frequent location of gout. Inflammatory changes are present, such as hyperechoic thickened subcutaneous fat containing hypoechoic lines in the subcutaneous tissue. Bone erosions can be associated underneath the tophus. Extensor tendons may be surrounded by tophi.

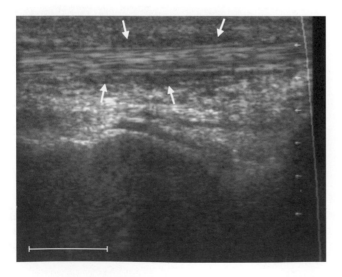

Fig. 439
The anterior tibial tendon (→) is surrounded by hypoechoic tissue in this patient with gout. No fibrous destruction was found.

Cystic Mass

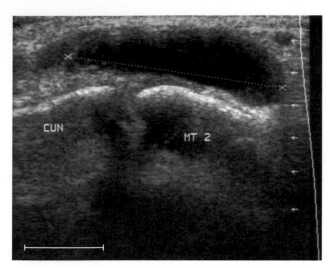

Fig. 440
An arthrosynovial cyst at the tarsometatarsal joint of the second toe in a sagittal plane.

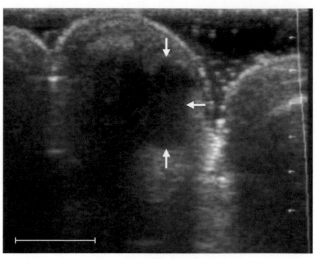

Fig. 441
A cyst (→) at the metatarsophalangeal joint of the fourth toe, seen in a transverse plane.

Cystic masses, such as arthrosynovial cysts or bursae, must be differentiated from Morton neuroma. Arthrosynovial cysts are anechoic lesions arising from a joint or a tendon sheath. Bursitis can develop medially to the first metatarsal head in hallux valgus deformity, corresponding to de novo bursitis, or more rarely between or underneath the metatarsal heads.

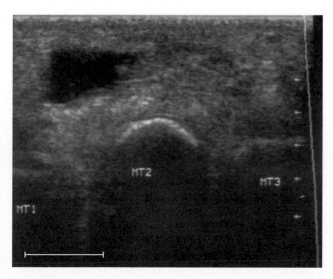

Fig. 442
A plantar, thick-walled de novo bursitis in the hypodermis centered on the second metatarsal head in a transverse scan.

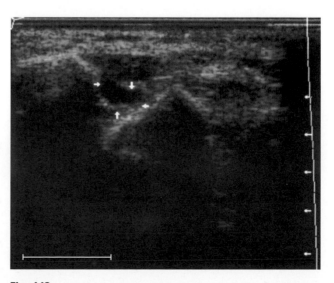

Fig. 443
Bursitis (→) in the intermetatarsal space, deep to the interosseous muscle.

Foot

Bone Injury

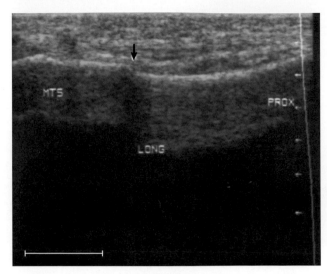

Fig. 444
A stress fracture of the fifth metatarsal bone shows cortical interruption (→) and a refraction shadow.

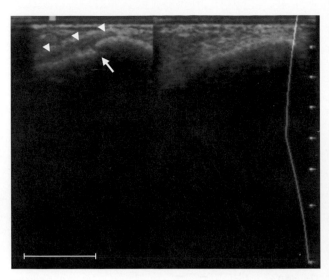

Fig. 445
A comparative study in a sagittal plane of the anterior border of both tali shows a stress fracture (→) with periosteal reaction on one side (▶) (**a** and **b**).

Painful bone lesions can be detected on ultrasound evaluation even without a history of acute trauma. Stress fractures are the most common in metatarsal bones. They usually occur at the second or third metatarsal. Ultrasound can detect stress fractures early, guided by palpation with the probe. The following anomalies can be detected: a periosteal reaction, showing as a hyperechoic band along the cortex; periosteal hemorrhage, in which the hyperechoic periosteum is elevated from the cortex by a hypoechoic band; and cortical interruption. Osteonecrosis and small fractures of tarsal bones can also be seen.

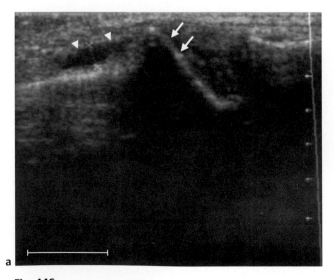

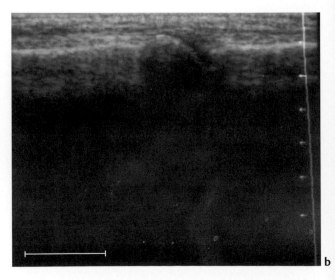

Fig. 446
A flattened metatarsal head (→) with associated joint effusion (▶) occurs in this young female with osteonecrosis of the metatarsal head (**a**). Comparative study (**b**).

Plantar Fasciitis

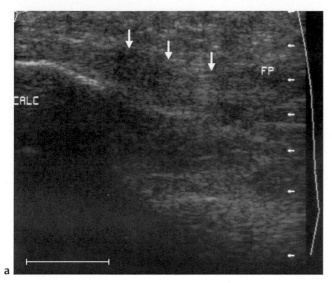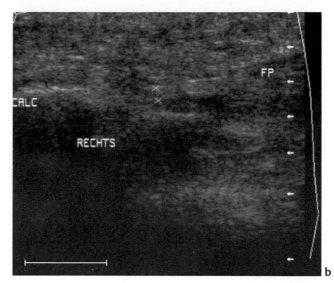

Fig. 447
A hypoechoic, indistinct plantar aponeurosis (→) at the anteroinferior border of the calcaneal tuberosity (**a**). Normal side for comparison (**b**).

Plantar fasciitis is an inflammation or partial rupture of the plantar fascia. Potential causes are mechanical and traumatic. In plantar fasciitis, the hyperechoic plantar aponeurosis can be thickened in comparison with the contralateral side. An enthesophyte can be seen as a hyperechoic band at the insertion on the calcaneum. The enthesophyte may be surrounded by a hypoechoic zone and accompanied by an acoustic shadow. De novo bursitis can be associated.

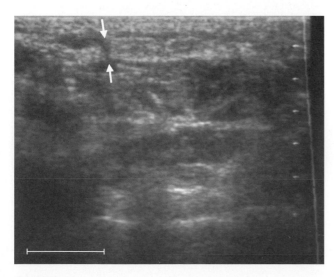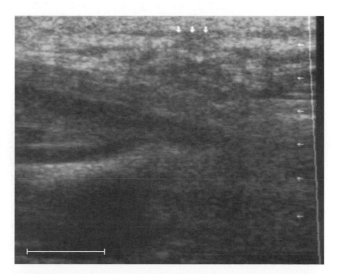

Fig. 448
A focal interruption of the plantar aponeurosis (→) superficial to the flexor digiti brevis muscle is seen on this transverse scan.

Fig. 449
A focal tender hypoechoic zone (→) is found in the plantar aponeurosis, indicating focal fasciitis after previous trauma.

Foot

Ledderhose Disease

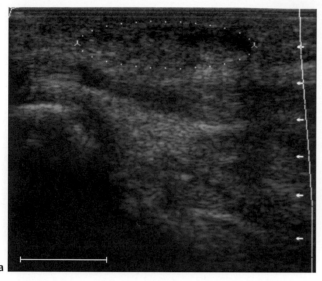
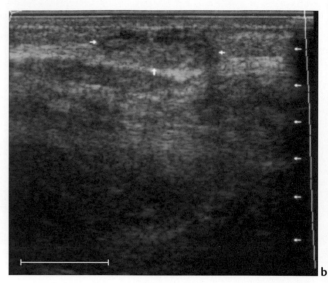

Fig. 450
An oval, heterogeneous, mixed hypoechoic and hyperechoic lesion (→) is found superficial to (**a**), or within (**b**) the plantar aponeurosis in patients with Ledderhose disease.

Plantar fibromatosis, or Ledderhose disease, affects 1–2% of the general population. The etiology is not clear. The age of onset is variable, the majority occurring in the fourth decade. It is a benign, but locally invasive neoplasm, consisting of a proliferation of fibroblasts in the plantar subcutaneous tissue of the foot. If incompletely resected, it can recur in a more aggressive form. Clinically, the lesions remain asymptomatic for a long period, and appear as one or more firm nodules. On ultrasound, the nodules are hypoechoic. The best method of evaluating these patients is MRI with gadolinium enhancement, to define the extent of infiltration and detect small satellite lesions prior to surgery.

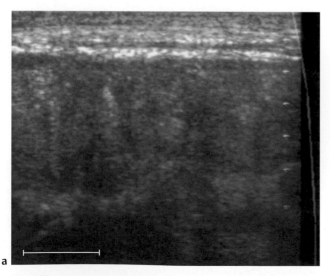
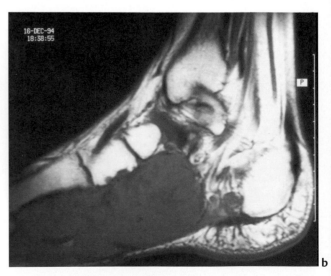

Fig. 451
A diffuse hypoechoic mass infiltrating the plantar soft tissues (**a**). The extent and invasive behavior of the lesion are better evaluated on a T$_1$-weighted MRI (**b**).

Morton Neuroma

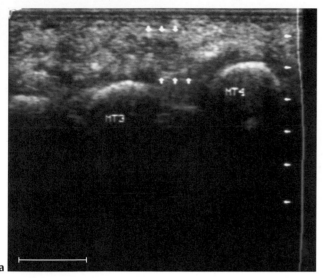

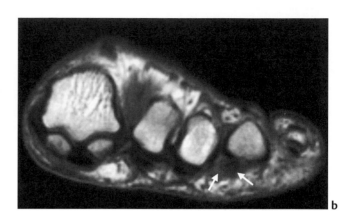

a　　　　　　　　　　　　　　　　　　　　　　　　　　　b

Fig. 452
A transverse scan of the plantar forefoot shows a neuroma (→) in the second metatarsal space as a hypoechoic mass (**a**). The corresponding T_1-weighted MRI after gadolinium administration confirms a hypointense, moderately enhanced, well delineated mass (→) (**b**).

Morton neuroma is a fibrous lesion of the plantar digital nerve found at the level of the metatarsal heads. It typically presents as a hypoechoic mass with an ovoid shape in the intermetatarsal space, deep to the interosseous muscles and distal to the intermetatarsal ligament. Sometimes the affected nerve is identified entering the mass at its proximal pole. Eighty percent of the patients affected are women, usually aged 25–50. On plain film, the distance between the metatarsal heads may be increased. Compression of the forefoot between the first and the fifth metatarsal head reveals the typical electrical pain. The third interdigital nerve is commonly involved.

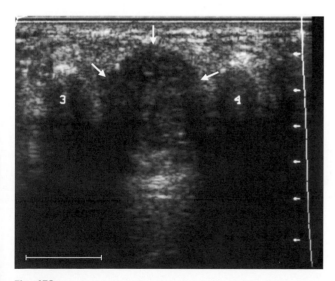

Fig. 453
A large Morton neuroma seen as a hypoechoic mass (→) between the third and fourth metatarsal head on this coronal plantar scan.

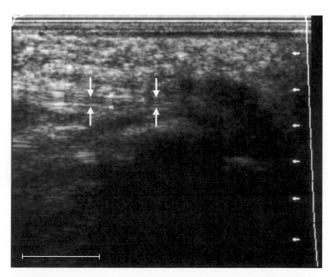

Fig. 454
The digital nerve (→) entering the neuroma is shown in its long axis, and measures 1.4 mm in diameter.

References

General Considerations

Castro W.H.M., Jerosch J., Schilgen M., Winkelmann W., The application of modern imaging methods in orthopedic surgery. Acta Orthop Belgica 1994, 60: 19–25

Chhem R.K., Kaplan P.A., Dussault R.G., Ultrasonography of the musculoskeletal system. Radiol Clin North Am 1994, 32: 275–289

Christensen R.A., Van Sonnenberg E., Casola G., Wittich G.R., Interventional Ultrasound in the musculoskeletal system. Radiol Clin North Am 1988, 26: 145–156

Fornage B.D., General ultrasound: musculoskeletal evaluation. Mittelsteadt C.A., Churchill Livingstone 1992: 1–57

Fornage B.D., Imagerie des parties molles de l'appareil locomoteur: échographie des parties molles. Getroa Opus 20, Sauramps Medical, 1993

Fornage B.D., Ultrasonography of muscles and tendons. Examination technique and atlas of normal anatomy of the extremities. Springer, 1987

Fornage B.D., Tassin G.B., Sonographic appearances of superficial soft tissue lipomas. J Clin Ultrasound 1991, 19: 215–220

Harcke H.T., Grissom L.E., Finkelstein M.S., Evaluation of the musculoskeletal system with sonography. AJR 1988, 150: 1253–1261

Hermann G., Yeh H.-C., Schwartz I., Computed tomography of soft-tissue lesions of the extremities, pelvic and shoulder girdles: sonographic and pathological correlations. Clin Radiol 1984, 35: 193–202

Howard C.B., Vinzberg A., Nyska M., Zirkin H., Aspiration of acute calcerous trochanteric bursitis using ultrasound guidance. J Clin Ultrasound 1993, 21: 45–47

James S.L., Bates B.T., Osternig L.R., Injuries to runners. Am J Sports Med 1978, 6: 40–50

Kaplan P.A., Matamoros A., Anderson J.C., Songoraphy of the musculoskeletal system. AJR 1990, 155: 237–245

Lenkey J.L., Skolnick M.L., Slasky B.S., Campbell W.L., Evaluation of the lower extremities. J Clin Ultrasound 1981, 9: 413–416

O'Keeffe D., Mamtora H., Ultrasound in clinical orthopaedics. J Bone Joint Surg 1992, 74-B: 488–94

Ralls P.W., Sonography in Rheumatology. Clin Rheumatol 1983, 9: 443–451

Resnick D., and Niwayana G., Diagnosis of bone and joint disorders. Saunders, 2nd Edition, 1988

Schlesinger A.E., Hernandez R.J., Diseases of the musculoskeletal system in children: imaging with CT, sonography, and MR. AJR 1992, 158: 729–741

Van Holsbeeck M., Introcaso J.H., Musculoskeletal ultrasonography. Radiol Clin North Am. 1992, 30: 907–925

Van Holsbeeck M., Introcaso J.H., Musculoskeletal ultrasound. Mosby Year Book, 1991

Vincent L.M., Ultrasound of soft tissue abnormalities of the extremities. Radiol Clin North Am 1988, 26: 131–144

Wilson D.J., Ultrasonic imaging of soft tissues. Clin Radiol 1989, 40: 341–342

Yeh H-C., Rabinowitz J.G., Ultrasonography of the extremities and pelvic girdle and correlation with computed tomography. Radiology 1982, 143: 519–525

Technical Aspects

Bloch J.G., Les explorations ultrasoniques de l'os, aspects fondamentaux et perspectives d'utilisation dans l'ostéoporose. Rev Rhum 1993, 60: 913–918

Laing F.C., Kurtz A.B., The importance of ultrasonic side-lobe artifacts. Radiology 1982, 145: 763–768

Parker K.J., Lerner R.M., Waag R.C., Attenuation of ultrasound: magnitude and frequency dependence for tissue characterization. Radiology 1984, 153: 785–788

Roux C., Lemonnier E., Kolta S., Charpentier E., Dougados M., Amor B., Viens Bitker C., Atténuation des ultrasons au calcanéum et densités osseuses. Rev Rhum 1993, 60: 897–906

Seltzer S.E., Finberg H.J., Weissman B.N, Arthrosonography-Technique, Sonographic Anatomy and Pathology. Invest Radiol 1980, 15: 19–28

Ziskin M.C., Thickman D.I., Goldenberg N.J., Lapayowker M.S., Becker J.M., The comet tail artifact. J Ultrasound Med 1982, 1: 1–7

Muscle

Amendola M.A., Glazer G.M., Agha F.P., Francis I.R., Weatherbee L., Martel W., Myositis ossificans circumscripta: computed tomographic diagnosis. Radiology 1983, 149: 775–779

Aspelin P., Pettersson H., Sigurjonsson S., Nilsson I.M., Ultrasonographic examinations of muscle hematomas in hemophiliacs. Acta Radiol Diagn 1984, 25: 513–516

Auerbach D.N., Bowen A.D., Sonography of leg in posterior compartment syndrome. AJR 1981, 136: 407–408

Brahim F., Zaccardelli W., Ultrasound measurement of the anterior leg compartment. Am J Sports Med 1986, 14: 300–302

Coelho J.C.U., Sigel B., Ryva J.C., Machi J., Renigers S.A., B-mode sonography of blood clots. J Clin Ultrasound 1982, 10: 323–327

Derchi L.E., Balconi G., De Flaviis L., Oliva A., Rosso F., Sonographic appearances of hemangiomas of skeletal muscle. J Ultrasound Med 1989, 8: 263–267

Fornage B.D., Eftekhari F., Sonographic diagnosis of myositis ossificans. J Ultrasound Med 1989, 8: 463–466

Fornage B.D., Nerot C., Sonographic diagnosis of rhabdomyolysis. J Clin Ultrasound 1986, 14: 389–392

Fornage B.D., Touche D.H., Segal P., Rifkin M.D., Ultrasonography in the evaluation of muscular trauma. J Ultrasound Med 1983, 2: 549–554

Giron J., Senac J.P., Myosite circonscrite hyperaigüe, pseudomaligne. J Radiol 1985, 66: 151–156

Giyanani V.L., Grozinger K.T., Gerlock A.J., Mirfakhraee M., Husbands H.S., Calf hematoma mimicking thrombophlebitis: sonographic and computed tomographic appearance. Radiology 1985, 154: 779–781

Goldman A.B., Myositis ossificans circumscripta: a benign lesion with a malignant differential diagnosis. AJR 1976, 126: 32–40

References

Graif M., Martinovitz U., Strauss S., Heim M., Itzchak Y., Sonographic localization of hematomas in hemophilic patients with positive iliopsoas sign. AJR 1987, 148: 121–123

Heckmatt J.Z., Pier N., Dubowitz V., Assessment of quadriceps femoris muscle atrophy and hypertrophy in neuromuscular disease in children. J Clin Ultrasound 1988, 16: 177–181

Heckmatt J.Z., Pier N., Dubowitz V., Measurement of quadriceps muscle thickness and subcutaneous tissue thickness in normal children by real-time ultrasound imaging. J Clin Ultrasound 1988, 16: 171–176

Kaplan G.N., Ultrasonic appearance of rhabdomyolysis. AJR 1980, 134: 375–377

Kirkpatrick J.S., Koman L.A., Rovere G.D., The role of ultrasound in the early diagnosis of myositis ossificans. Am J Sports Med 1987, 15: 179–181

Kramer F.L., Kurtz A.B., Rubin C., Goldberg B.B., Ultrasound appearance of myositis ossificans. Skeletal Radiol 1979, 4: 19–20

Laine H., Harjula A., Peltokallio P., Varstela E., Real time sonography to diagnose soft-tissue sports injuries. Lancet, 1984, 7: 55

Lamminen A.E., Hekali P.E., Tiula E., Suramo I., Korhola O.A., Acute rhabdomyolysis: evaluation with magnetic resonance imaging compared with computed tomography and ultrasonography. Br J Radiol 1989, 62: 326–331

Lamminen A., Jääskeläinen J., Rapola J., Suramo I., High-frequency ultrasonography of skeletal muscle in children with neuromuscular disease. J Ultrasound Med 1988, 7: 505–509

Lehto M., Alanen A., Healing of a muscle trauma: correlation of sonographical and histological findings in an experimental study in rats. J Ultrasound Med 1987, 6: 425–429

Martens M.A., Backaert M., Vermaut G., Mulier J.C., Chronic leg pain in athletes due to a recurrent compartment syndrome. Am J Sports Med 1984, 12: 148–151

Ogilvie-Harris D.J., Hons Ch.B., Fornasier V.L., Pseudomalignant myositis ossificans: heterotopic new-bone formation without a history of trauma. J Bone Joint Surg 1980, 62: 1274–1283

Paterson D.C., Myositis ossificans circumscripta. J Bone Joint Surg 1970, 52: 296–301

Peck R.J., Metreweli C., Early myositis ossificans: a new echographic sign. Clin Radiol 1988, 39: 586–588

Quillin S.P., McAlister W.H., Rapidly progressive pyomyositis. J Ultrasound Med 1991, 10: 181–184

Roy C., Challan-Belval P., Myosite ossifiante non traumatique. Aspects échographique et scanographique. J Radiol 1985, 66: 473–475

van Sonnenberg E., Wittich G.R., Casola G., Cabrera O.A., Gosink B.B., Resnick D.L., Sonography of thigh abscess: detection, diagnosis, and drainage. AJR 1987, 149: 769–772

Vukanovic S., Hauser H., Curati W.L., Myonecrosis induced by drug overdose: pathogenesis, clinical aspects and radiological manifestations. Eur J Radiol 1983, 3: 314–318

Wicks J.D., Silver T.M., Bree R.L., Gray scale features of hematomas: an ultrasonic spectrum. AJR 1978, 131: 977–980

Yaghmai I., Myositis ossificans: diagnostic value of arteriography. AJR 1977, 128: 811–816

Yousefzadeh D.K., Schumann E.M., Mulligan G.M., Bosworth D.E., Young C.S., Pringle K.C., The role of imaging modalities in diagnosis and management of pyomyositis. Skeletal Radiol 1982, 8: 285–289

Tendon

Baker K.S., Gilula L.A., The current role of tenography and bursography. AJR 1990, 154: 129–133

Bouffard J.A., Eyler W.R., Introcaso J.H., van Holsbeeck M., Sonography of tendons. Ultrasound Quarterly 1993, 11: 259–286

Chevremont M., Cytologie et histologie, Desoer, 3rd edition, 1975, 553

Crass J.R., van de Vegte G.L., Harkavy L.A., Tendon echogenicity: ex vivo study. Radiology 1988, 167: 499–501

Dillehay G.L., Deschler T., Rogers L.F., Neiman H.L., Hendrix R.W., The ultrasonographic characterization of tendons. Invest Radiol 1984, 19: 338–341

Fornage B.D., Rifkin M.D., Ultrasound examination of tendons. Radiol Clin North Am 1988, 26: 87–107

Fornage B.D., Soft-tissue changes in the hand in rheumatoid arthritis: evaluation with US. Radiology 1989, 173: 735–737

Fornage B.D., The hypoechoic normal tendon a pitfall. J Ultrasound Med 1987, 6: 19–22

Jeffrey R.B., Laing F.C., Schechter W.P., Markison R.E., Barton R.M., Acute suppurative tenosynovitis of the hand: diagnosis with US. Radiology 1987, 162: 741–742

Morgan J., McCarty D.J, Tendon ruptures in patients with systemic lupus erythematosus treated with corticosteroids. Arthritis Rheum 1974, 17: 1033–1036

Ligament

De Flaviis L., Nessi R., Leonardi M., Ulivi M., Dynamic ultrasonography of capsulo-ligamentous knee joint traumas. J Clin Ultrasound 1988, 16: 487–492

Frank C., Amiel D., Akeson W.H., Healing of the medial collateral ligament of the knee: a morphological and biochemical assessment in rabbits. Acta Orthop Scand 1983, 54: 917–923

Hastings D.E., Knee ligament instability-a rational anatomical classification. Clin Orthop 1986, 208: 104–107

Hastings D.E., The non-operative management of collateral ligament injuries of the knee joint. Clin Orthop 1980, 147: 22–28

Laws G., Walton M., Fibroblastic healing of grade II ligament injuries. J Bone Joint Surg 1988, 70-B: 390–396

Bone

Abernethy L.J., Lee Y.C.P., Orth M. Ch., Cole W.G., Ultrasound localization of subperiosteal abscesses in children with late-acute osteomyelitis. J Pediatr Orthop 1993, 13: 766–768

Abiri M.M., Kirpekar M., Ablow R.C., Osteomyelitis: detection with US. Radiology 1988, 169: 795–797

Abiri M.M., Kirpekar M., Ablow R.C., Osteomyelitis: detection with US. Radiology 1989, 172: 509–511

Cartoni C., Capua A., Damico C., Potente G., Aspergillus osteomyelitis of the rib: sonographic diagnosis. J Clin Ultrasound 1992, 20: 217–220

Graif M., Stahl-Kent V., Ben-Ami T., Strauss S., Amit Y., Itzchak Y., Sonographic detection of occult bone fractures. Pediatr Radiol 1988, 18: 383–385

Hammond I., Unsuspected humeral head fracture diagnosed by ultrasound. J Ultrasound Med 1991, 10: 422

Mahaisavariya B., Suibnugarn C., Mairiang E., Saengnipanthkul S., Laupattarakasem W., Kosuwon W., Ultrasound for closed femoral nailing. J Clin Ultrasound 1991, 19: 393–397

Malghem J., Vande Berg B., Noël H., Maldague B., Benign osteochondromas and exostotic chondrosarcomas: evaluation of cartilage cap thickness by ultrasound. Skeletal Radiol 1992, 21: 33–37

Mukuno D.H., Lee T.G., Watanabe A.S., McIff E.B., Aneurysmal bone cyst presenting as a pelvic mass on sonographic examination. J Ultrasoung Med 1986, 5: 215–216

Nath A.K., Sethu A.U., Use of ultrasound in osteomyelitis. Br J Radiol 1992, 65: 649–652

Steiner G.M., Sprigg A., The value of ultrasound in the assessment of bone. Br J Radiol 1992, 65: 589–593

Young J.W.R., Kostrubiak I.S., Resnik C.S., Paley D., Sonographic evaluation of bone production at the distraction site in Ilizarov limb-lengthening procedures. AJR 1990, 154: 125–128

Joint-Bursa

Cooperberg P.L., Tsang I., Truelove L, Knickerbocker J., Gray scale ultrasound in the evaluation of rheumatoid arthritis of the knee. Radiology 1978, 126: 759–763

De Flaviis L., Nessi R., Del Bo P., Calori G., Balconi G., High-Resolution ultrasonography of wrist ganglia. J Clin Ultrasound 1987, 15: 17–22

De Flaviis L., Nessi R., Leonardi M., Ulivi M., Dynamic ultrasonography of capsulo-ligamentous knee joint traumas. J Clin Ultrasound 1988, 16: 487–492

Fedullo L.M., Bonakdarpour A., Moyer R.A., Tourtellotte C.D., Giant synovial cysts. Skeletal Radiol 1984, 12: 90–96

Gilsanz V., Bernstein B.H., Joint calcification following intra-articular corticosteroid therapy. Radiology 1984, 151: 647–649

Grassi W., Tittarelli E., Pirani O., Avaltroni D., Cervini C., Ultrasound examination of metacarpophalangeal joints in rheumatoid arthritis. Scand J Rheumatol 1993, 22: 243–247

Hammer M., Mielke H., Wagener P., Schwarzrock R., Giebel G., Sonography and NMR imaging in rheumatoid gonarthritis. Scand J Rheumatol 1986, 15: 157–164

Janus C., Hermann G., Enlargement of the iliopsoas bursa: unusual cause of cystic mass on pelvic sonogram. J Clin Ultrasound 1982, 10: 133–135

Kaufman R.A., Towbin R.B., Babcock D.S., Crawford A.H., Arthrosonography in the diagnosis of pigmented villonodular synovitis. AJR 1982, 139: 396–398

Lerais J.M., Baudrillard J.C., Durot J.F., Segal Ph., Tellart M.O., Wallays C., Auquier F., Toubas O., Petit J., Kystes synoviaux de topographie inhabituelle: deux observations et revue de la littérature. J Radiol 1986, 67: 201–207

Moss G.D., Dishuk W., Ultrasound diagnosis of osteochondromatosis of the popliteal fossa. J Clin Ultrasound 1984, 12: 232–233

Pellman E., Kumari S., Greenwald R., Rheumatoid iliopsoas bursitis presenting as unilateral leg edema. J Rheumatol 1986, 13: 197–200

Rao A.S., Vigorita V.J., Pigmented villonodular synovitis (giant-cell tumor of the tendon sheath and synovial membrane). J Bone Joint Surg 1984, 66-A: 76–94

Shepherd J.R., Helms C.A., Atypical popliteal cyst due to lateral synovial herniation. Radiology 1981, 140: 66

Spiegel T.M., King W., Weiner S.R., Paulus H.E., Measuring disease activity: comparison of joint tenderness, swelling, and ultrasonography in rheumatoid arthritis. Arthritis Rheum 1987, 30: 1283–1288

Sureda D., Quiroga S., Arnal C., Boronat M., Andreu J., Casas L., Juvenile rheumatoid arthritis of the knee: evaluation with US. Radiology 1994, 190: 403–406

Cartilage

Aisen A.M., McCune W.J., MacGuire A., Carson P.L., Silver T.M., Jafri S.Z., Martel W., Sonographic evaluation of the cartilage of the knee. Radiology 1984, 153: 781–784

Martino F., Ettorre G.C., Angelelli G., Macarini L., Patella V., Moretti B., D'Amore M., Cantatore F.P., Validity of echographic evaluation of cartilage in gonarthrosis. Preliminary report. Clin Rheumatol 1993, 12: 178–183

McCune W.J., Dedrick D.K., Aisen A.M., MacGuire A., Sonographic evaluation of osteoarthritic femoral condylar cartilage: correlation with operative findings. Clin Orthop 1990, 254: 230–235

Selby B., Richardson M.L., Montana M.A., Teitz C.C., Larson R.V., Mack L.A., High resolution sonography of the menisci of the knee. Invest Radiol 1986, 21: 332–335

Selby B., Richardson M.L., Nelson B.D., Graney D.O., Mack L.A., Sonography in the detection of meniscal injuries of the knee: evaluation in cadavers. AJR 1987, 149: 549–553

Vessel

Alanen A., Kormano M., Correlation of the echogenicity and structure of clotted blood. J Ultrasound Med 1985, 4: 421–425

Aronen H.J., Pamilo M., Suoranta H.T., Suramo I., Sonography in differential diagnosis of deep venous thrombosis of the leg. Acta Radiol 1987, 28: 457–459

Dauzat M.M., Laroche J.P., Charras C., Blin B., Domingo-Faye M.M., Sainte-Luce P., Domergue A., Lopez F.M., Janbon C., Real-time B-Mode ultrasonography for better specifity in the noninvasive diagnosis of deep venous thrombosis. J Ultrasound Med 1986, 5: 625–631

Davis R.P., Neiman H.L., Yao J.S.T., Bergan J.J., Ultrasound scan in diagnosis of peripheral aneurysms. Arch Surg 1977, 112: 55–58

Greenspan A., McGahan J.P., Vogelsang P., Szabo R.M., Imaging strategies in the evaluation of soft-tissue hemangiomas of the extremities: correlation of the findings of plain radiography, angiography, CT, MRI, and ultrasonography in 12 histologically proven cases. Skeletal Radiol 1992, 21: 11–18

Longo J.M., Rodriguez-Cabello J., Bilbao J.I., Aquerreta J.D., Ruza M., Mansilla F., Popliteal vein thrombosis and popliteal artery compression complicating fibular osteochondroma: ultrasound diagnosis. J Clin Ultrasound 1990, 18: 507–509

Mitchell D.G., Needleman L., Bezzi M., Goldberg B.B., Kurtz A.B., Pennell R.G., Rifkin M.D., Vilaro M., Baltarowich O.H., Femoral artery pseudoaneurysm: diagnosis with conventional duplex and color doppler US. Radiology 1987, 165: 687–690

Neiman H.L., Yao J.S.T., Silver T.M., Gray-scale ultrasound diagnosis of peripheral arterial aneurysms. Radiology 1979, 130: 413–416

References

O'Keeffe F., Fornage B.D., Engainement bilatéral de la veine saphène interne chez un patient atteint de lymphome. J Radiol 1990, 71: 369–371

Raghavendra B.N., Horii S.C., Hilton S., Subramanyam B.R., Rosen R.J., Lam S., Deep venous thrombosis: detection by probe compression of veins. J Ultrasound Med 1986, 5: 89–95

Ritchie D.A., Hill D., Fullarton G.M., Calvert M.H., Ultrasound diagnosis of profunda femoris pseudo-aneurysm following nail-plate fixation of a transcervical femoral fracture. Br J Radiol 1987, 60: 502–504

Sarti D.A., Louie J.S., Lindstrom R.R., Nies K., London J., Ultrasonic diagnosis of a popliteal artery aneurysm. Radiology 1976, 121: 707–708

Silver T.M., Washburn R.L., Stanley J.C., Gross W.S., Gray scale ultrasound evaluation of popliteal artery aneurysms. AJR 1977, 129: 1003–1006

Wales L.R., Azose A.A., Saphenous varix: ultrasonic diagnosis. J Ultrasound Med 1985, 4: 143–145

Weinberger J., Marks S.J., Gaul J.J., Goldman B., Schanzer H., Jacobson J., Dikman S., Atherosclerotic plaque at the carotid artery bifurcation. J Ultrasound Med 1987, 6: 363–366

Nerve

Burkitt H.G., Young B., Heath J.W., Functional histology: a text and colour atlas. Churchill Livingstone, Third Edition 1993: 126–127

Cantos-Melian B., Arriaza-Loureda R., Aisa-Varela P., Tibialis posterior nerve schwannoma mimicking Achilles tendinitis: ultrasonographic diagnosis. J Clin Ultrasound 1990, 18: 671–673

Chinn D.H., Filly R.A., Callen P.W., Unusual ultrasonographic appearance of a solid schwannoma. J Clin Ultrasound 1982, 10: 243–245

Fornage B.D., Peripheral nerves of the extremities: imaging with US. Radiology 1988, 167: 179–182

Fornage B.D., Touche D.H., Rifkin M.D., Small-parts real-time sonography: a new "water path". J Ultrasound Med 1984, 3: 355–357

Hoddick W.K., Callen P.W., Filly R.A., Mahony B.S., Edwards M.B., Ultrasound evaluation of benign sciatic nerve sheath tumors. J Ultrasound Med 1984, 3: 505–507

Hughes D.G., Wilson D.J., Ultrasound appearances of peripheral nerve tumors. Br J Radiol 1986, 59: 1041–1043

Redd R.A., Peters V.J., Emery S.F., Branch H.M., Rifkin M.D., Morton Neuroma: sonographic evaluation. Radiology 1989, 171: 415–417

Reuter K.L., Raptopoulos V., DeGirolami U., Akins C.M., Ultrasonography of a plexiform neurofibroma of the popliteal fossa. J Ultrasound Med 1982, 1: 209–211

Skin and Subcutaneous Tissue

Behan M., Kazam E., The echographic characteristics of fatty tissues and tumors. Radiology 1978, 129: 143–151

Bernardino M.E., Jing B.S., Thomas J.L., Lindell M.M., Zornoza J., The extremity soft-tissue lesion: a comparative study of ultrasound computed tomography and xeroradiography. Radiology 1981, 139: 53–59

Braunstein E.M., Silver T.M., Martel W., Jaffe M., Ultrasonographic diagnosis of extremity masses. Skeletal Radiol 1981, 6: 157–163

Cole G.W., Handler S.J., Burnett K., The ultrasonic evaluation of skin thickness in scleroderma. J Clin Ultrasound 1981, 9: 501–503

Fornage B.D., Deshayes J.L., Ultrasound of normal skin. J Clin Ultrasound 1986, 14: 619–622

Fornage B.D., Nerot C., Sonographic diagnosis of tuberculoid leprosy. J Ultrasound Med 1987, 6: 105–107

Fornage B.D., Tassin G.B., Sonographic appearances of superficial soft tissue lipomas. J Clin Ultrasound 1991, 19: 215–220

Konno K., Ishida H., Morikawa P., Uno A., Niizawa M., Naganuma H., Masamune O., Niizawa M., Sonographic appearance of extensive subcutaneous calcification. J Clin Ultrasound 1992, 20: 415–418

Nessi R., Betti R., Bencini P.L., Crosti C., Blanc M., Uslenghi C., Ultrasonography of nodular and infiltrative lesions of the skin and subcutaneous tissues. J Clin Ultrasound 1990, 18: 103–109

Pamilo M., Soiva M., Lavast E.M., Real-time ultrasound, axillary mammography, and clinical examination in the detection of axillary lymph node metastases in breast cancer patients. J Ultrasound Med 1989, 8: 115–120

Sandler M.A., Alpern M.B., Madrazo B.L., Gitschlag K.F., Inflammatory lesions of the groin: ultrasonic evaluation. Radiology 1984, 151: 747–750

Tiliakos N., Morales A.R., Wilson C.H., Use of ultrasound in identifying tophaceous versus rheumatoid nodules. Arthritis Rheum 1982, 25: 478–479

Foreign Body

Anderson M.A., Newmeyer W.L., Kilgore E.S., Diagnosis and treatment of retained foreign bodies in the hand. Am J Surg 1982, 144: 63–65

Banerjee B., Das R.K., Sonographic detection of foreign bodies of the extremities. Br J Radiol 1991, 64: 107–112

De Flaviis L., Scaglione P., Del Bö P., Nessi R., Detection of foreign bodies in soft tissues: experimental comparison of ultrasonography and xeroradiography. J Trauma 1988, 28: 400–404

Donaldson J.S., Radiographic imaging of foreign bodies in the hand. Hand Clin 1991, 7: 125–134

Fornage B.D., Peroperative sonographic localization of a migrated transosseous stabilizing wire in the hand. J Ultrasound Med 1987, 6: 471–473

Fornage B.D., Schernberg F.L., Sonographic diagnosis of foreign bodies of the distal extremities. AJR 1986, 147: 567–569

Fornage B.D., Schernberg F.L., Sonographic preoperative localization of a foreign body in the hand. J Ultrasound Med 1987, 6: 217–219

Gooding G.A.W., Hardiman T., Sumers M., Stess R., Graf P., Grunfeld C., Sonography of the hand and foot in foreign body detection. J Ultrasound Med 1987, 6: 441–447

Gordon D., Non-metallic foreign bodies. Br J Radiol 1985, 58: 574

Howard C.B., Nyska M., Mellor I., Leiberman N., Mozes G., Sonographic underestimation of the size of a foreign body. J Clin Ultrasound 1992, 20: 412–414

Kobs J.K., Hansen A.R., Keefe B., A retained wooden foreign body in the foot detected by ultrasonography. J Bone Joint Surg 1992, 74-A: 296–298

Little C.M., Parker M.G., Callowich M.C., Sartori J.C., The ultrasonic detection of soft tissue foreign bodies. Invest Radiol 1986, 21: 275–277

Pascal-Suisse P., Castinel B., Peyron J.P., Vergne R., Pringot J., Textile foreign bodies: echotomographic and computed tomography of five cases. J Belge Radiol 1982, 65: 355–361

Pery M., Rosenberger A., Kaftori J.K., Ultrasonographic detection of plastic materials in various organs of the human body. J Clin Ultrasound 1989, 17: 489–495

Wendell B.A., Athey P.A., Ultrasonic appearance of metallic foreign bodies in parenchymal organs. J Clin Ultrasound 1981, 9: 133–135

Ziskin M.C., Thickman D.I., Goldenberg N.J., Lapayowker M.S., Becker J.M., The comet tail artifact. J Ultrasound Med 1982, 1: 1–7

Shoulder

Ahovuo J., Paavolainen P., Homström T., Ultrasonography of the tendons of the shoulder. Eur J Radiol 1989, 9: 17–21

Bartolozzi A., Andreychik D., Ahmad S., Determinants of outcome in the treatment of rotator cuff disease. Clin Orthop 1994, 308: 90–97

Bassett R.W., Cofield R.H., Acute tears of the rotator cuff. Clin Orthop 1983, 175: 18–24

Beltran J., Gray L.A., Bools J.C., Zuelzer W., Weis L.D., Unverferth L.J., Rotator cuff lesions of the shoulder: evaluation by direct sagittal CT arthrography. Radiology 1986, 160: 161–165

Brandt T.D., Cardone B.W., Grant T.H., Post M., Weiss C.A., Rotator cuff sonography: a reassessment. Radiology 1989, 173: 323–327

Brasseur J.L., Lazennec J.Y., Tardieu M., Richard O., Roger B., Grenier Ph., Echographie dynamique de l'épaule dans le conflit antéro-supérieur. Rev Im Med 1994, 6: 629–631

Bretzke C.A., Crass J.R., Craig E.V., Feinberg S.B., Ultrasonography of the rotator cuff: normal and pathologic anatomy. Invest Radiol 1985, 20: 311–315

Burk D.L., Jr., Karasick D., Kurtz A.B., Mitchell D.G., Rifkin M.D., Miller C.L., Levy D.W., Fenlin J.M., Bartolozzi A.R., Rotator cuff tears: prospective comparison of MR imaging with arthrography, sonography, and surgery. AJR 1989, 153: 87–92

Cofield R.H., Current concepts review: rotator cuff disease of the shoulder. J Bone and Joint Surg 1985, 67-A: 974–979

Collins R.A., Gristina A.G., Carter R.E., Webb L.X., Voytek A., Ultrasonography of the shoulder: static and dynamic imaging. Orthop Clin North Am 1987, 18: 351–360

Cone R.O., Danzig L., Resnick D., Goldman A.B., The bicipital groove: radiographic, anatomic, and pathologic study. AJR 1983, 141: 781–788

Conrad M.R., Nelms B.A., Empty bicipital groove due to rupture and retraction of the biceps tendon. J Ultrasound Med 1990, 9: 231–233

Crass J.R., Craig E.V., Feinberg S.B., Clinical significance of sonographic findings in the abnormal but intact rotator cuff: a preliminary report. J Clin Ultrasound 1988, 16: 625–634.

Crass J.R., Craig E.V., Feinberg S.B., Sonography of the postoperative rotator cuff. AJR 1986, 146: 561–564

Crass J.R., Craig E.V., Feinberg S.B., The hyperextended internal rotation view in rotator cuff ultrasonography. J Clin Ultrasound 1987, 15: 416–420

Crass J.R., Craig E.V., Feinberg S.B., Utrasonography of rotator cuff tears: a review of 500 diagnostic studies. J Clin Ultrasound 1988, 16: 313–327

Crass J.R., Craig E.V., Thompson R.C., Feinberg S.B., Ultrasonography of the rotator cuff: surgical correlation. J Clin Ultrasound 1984, 12: 487–492

Drakeford M.K., Quinn M.J., Simpson S.L., Pettine K.A., A comparative study of ultrasonography and arthrography in evaluation of the rotator cuff. Clin Orthop 1990, 253: 118–122

Farin P.U., Jaroma H., Harju A., Soimakallio S., Shoulder impingement syndrome sonographic evaluation. Radiology 1990, 176: 845–849

Furtschegger A., Resch H., Value of ultrasonography in preoperative diagnosis of rotator cuff tears and postoperative follow-up. Eur J Radiol 1988, 8: 69–75

Hall F.M., Sonography of the shoulder. Radiology 1989, 173: 310

Hawkins R.J., Abrams J.S., Impingement syndrome in the absence of rotator cuff tear (stages 1 and 2). Orthop Clin North Am 1987, 18: 373–382

Hodler J., Fretz C.J., Terrier F., Gerber C., Rotator cuff tears: correlation of sonographic and surgical findings. Radiology 1988, 169: 791–794

Jobe F.W., Jobe C.M., Painful athletic injuries of the shoulder. Clin Orthop 1983, 173: 117–124

Katthagen B.D., Ultrasonography of the shoulder: technique, anatomy, pathology. Thieme 1990

Kay J., Benson C.B., Lester S., Corson J.M., Pinkus G.S., Lazarus J.M., Owen W.F., Jr, Utility of high-resolution ultrasound for the diagnosis of dialysis-related amyloidosis. Arthritis Rheum 1992, 35: 926–932

Kilcoyne R.F., Matsen F.A., Rotator cuff tear measurement by arthropneumo-tomography. AJR 1983, 140: 315–318

Kurol M., Rahme H., Hilding S., Sonography for diagnosis of rotator cuff tear: comparison with observations at surgery in 58 shoulders. Acta Orthop Scand 1991, 62: 465–567

Lanzer W.L., Clinical aspects of shoulder injuries. Radiol Clin North Am 1988, 26: 157–160

Lawson T.L., Middleton W.D., MRI and ultrasound evaluation of the shoulder. Acta Orthop Belg 1991, 57: 62–69

Lyons A.R, Tomlinson J.E., Clinical diagnosis of tears of the rotator cuff. J Bone Joint Surg 1992, 74-B: 414–415

Mack L.A., Matsen F.A., Kilcoyne R.F., Davies P.K., Sickler M.E., US evaluation of the rotator cuff. Radiology 1985, 157: 205–209

Mack L.A., Nyberg D.A., Matsen F.R., Kilcoyne R.F., Harvey D., Sonography of the postoperative shoulder. AJR 1988, 150: 1089–1093

Mack L.A., Nyberg D.A., Matsen F.A., Sonographic evaluation of the rotator cuff. Radiol Clin North Am 1988, 26: 161–177

Middleton W.D., Status of rotator cuff sonography. Radiology 1989, 173: 307–309

Middleton W.D., Ultrasonography of the shoulder. Radiol Clin North Am 1992, 30: 927–940

Middleton W.D., Edelstein G., Reinus W.R., Melson G.L., Murphy W.A., Ultrasonography of the rotator cuff: technique and normal anatomy. J Ultrasound Med 1984, 3: 549–551

Middleton W.D., Edelstein G., Reinus W.R., Melson G.L., Totty W.G., Murphy W.A., Sonographic detection of rotator cuff tears. AJR 1985, 144: 349–353

Middleton W.D., Reinus W.R., Melson G.L., Totty W.G., Murphy W.A., Pitfalls of rotator cuff sonography. AJR 1986, 146: 555–560

Middleton W.D., Reinus W.R., Totty W.G., Melson C.L., Murphy W.A., Ultrasonographic evaluation of the rotator

References

cuff and biceps tendon. J Bone Joint Surg 1986, 68-A: 440–450

Middleton W.D., Reinus W.R., Totty W.G., Melson G.L., Murphy W.A., US of the biceps tendon apparatus. Radiology 1985, 157: 211–215

Miller C.L., Karasick D., Kurtz A.B., Fenlin J.M., Limited sensitivity of ultrasound for the detection of rotator cuff tears. Skeletal Radiol 1989, 18: 179–183

Moseley H.F., Goldie I., The arterial pattern of the rotator cuff of the shoulder. J Bone Joint Surg 1963, 45-B: 780–789

Neer C.S., Anterior acromioplasty for the chronic impingement syndrome in the shoulder. J Bone Joint Surg 1972, 54-A: 41–50

Neer C.S., Impingement lesions. Clin Orthop 1983, 173: 70–77

Neviaser R.J, Ruptures of the rotator cuff. Orthop Clin North Am. 1987, 18: 387–394

Nevasier T.J., The role of the biceps tendon in the impingement syndrome. Orthop Clin North Am 1987, 18: 383–386

O'Donoghue D.H., Subluxing biceps tendon in the athlete. Clin Orthop 1982, 164: 26–29

Paavolainen P., Ahovuo J., Ultrasonography and arthrography in the diagnosis of tears of the rotator cuff. J Bone Joint Surg, 1994, 76-A: 335–340

Peetrons Ph., Delmotte S., Stehman M., Peetrons A., Lésions de la coiffe des rotateurs: apport spécifique de l'échographie. Acta Orthop Belg 1986, 52: 703–716

Peetrons P., Echographie de l'épaule. Feuillets Radiol 1987, 27: 299–302

Petersson C.J., Gentz C.F., Ruptures of the supraspinatus tendon: the significance of distally pointing acromioclavicular osteophytes. Clin Orthop 1983, 174: 143–148

Petersson C.J., Spontaneous medical dislocation of the tendon of the long biceps brachii. Clin Orthop 1986, 211: 224–227

Post M., Silver R., Singh M., Rotator cuff tear: diagnosis and treatment. Clin Orthop 1983, 173: 78–91

Resnick D., Shoulder arthrography. Radiol Clin North Am 1981, 19: 243–253

Sarrafian S.K., Gross and functional anatomy of the shoulder. Clin Orthop 1983, 173: 11–19

Seeger L.L., Diagnostic imaging of the shoulder. Williams and Wilkins 1992

Seltzer S.E., Finberg H.J., Weissman B.N., Kido D.K., Collier B.D., Arthrosonography: gray-scale ultrasound evaluation of the shoulder. Radiology 1979, 132: 467–468

Soble M.G., Kaye A.D., Guay R.C., Rotator cuff tear: clinical experience with sonographic detection. Radiology 1989, 173: 319–321

Van Holsbeeck M., Introcaso J., Sonography of the postoperative shoulder. AJR 1989, 152: 202

Vicens J.L., Flageat J., Eulry F., Pattin S., Doury P., Bursite de l'épaule au cours d'une polyarthrite rhumatoïde. J Radiol 1989, 70: 649–651

Vick W.C., Bell S.A., Rotator cuff tears: diagnosis with sonography. AJR 1990, 154: 121–123

Wolfgang G.L., Rupture of the musculotendinous cuff of the shoulder. Clin Orthop 1978, 134: 230–243

Elbow

Alnot J.Y., Boulate M., Les épicondylalgies, diagnostic et traitement. Ann Chir Main (Ann Hand Surg) 1993, 12: 5–11

Bennett J.B., Lateral and medial epicondylitis. Hand Clin 1994, 10: 157–163

Chard M.D., Cawston T.E., Riley G.P., Gresham G.A., Hazleman B.L., Rotator cuff degeneration and lateral epicondylitis: a comparative histological study. Ann Rheum Dis 1994, 53: 30–34

Doran A., Gresham G.A., Rushton N., Watson Ch., Tennis elbow: a clinicopathologic study of 22 cases followed for 2 years. Acta Orthop Scand 1990, 61: 535–538

Karasick D., Burk D.L., Gross G.W., Trauma to the elbow and forearm. Semin Roentgenol 1991, 26: 318–330

Lyons A.R., Porter K.M., Chondromatose synoviale post-traumatique du coude chez un enfant de 8 ans. Rev Chir Orthop 1993, 124–126

Markowitz R.I., Davidson R.S., Harty M.P., Bellah R.D., Hubbard A.M., Rosenberg H.K., Sonography of the elbow in infants and children. AJR 1992, 159: 829–833

Miles K.A., Lamont A.C., Ultrasonic demonstration of the elbow fat pads. Clin Radiol 1989, 40: 602–604

Nirschl R.P., Elbow tendinosis, tennis elbow. Clin Sports Med 1992, 11: 851–870

Paterson J.M.H., Roper B.A., Olecranon spur. J Hand Surg 1993, 18-B: 9–10

Rath A.M., Perez M., Mainguené C., Masquelet A.C., Chevrel J.P., Anatomic basis of the physiopathology of the epicondylalgias: a study of the deep branch of the radial nerve. Surg Radiol Anat 1993, 15: 15–19

- Regan W., Wold L.E., Coonrad R., Morrey B.F., Microscopic histopathology of chronic refractory lateral epicondylitis. Am J Sports Med 1992, 20: 746–749

Hand and Wrist

Andrén L., Eiken O., Arthrographic studies of wrist ganglions. J Bone Joint Surg 1971, 53-A: 299–302

Bianchi S., Abdelwahab I.F., Zwass A., Giacomello P., Ultrasonographic evaluation of wrist ganglia. Skeletal Radiol 1994, 23: 201–203

Buchberger W., Judmaier W., Birbamer G., Lener M., Schmidauer C., Carpal tunnel syndrome: diagnosis with high-resolution sonography. AJR 1992, 159: 793–798

Cardinal, E., Buckwalter K.A., Braunstein E.M., Mih A.D., Occult dorsal carpal ganglion: comparison of US and MR imaging. Radiology 1994, 193: 259–262

De Flaviis L., Scaglione P., Nessi R., Ventura R., Calori G., Ultrasonography of the hand in rheumatoid arthritis. Acta Radiol 1988, 29: 457–460

Fornage B.D., Glomus tumors in the fingers: diagnosis with US. Radiology 1988, 167: 183–185

Fornage B.D., Rifkin M.D., Ultrasound examination of the hand. Radiology 1986, 160: 853–854

Fornage B.D., Rifkin M.D., Ultrasound examination of the hand and foot. Radiol Clin North Am 1988, 26: 109–129

Fornage B.D., Schernberg F.L., Rifkin M.D., Touche D.H., Sonographic diagnosis of glomus tumor of the finger. J Ultrasound Med 1984, 3: 523–524

Fornage, B.D., Schernberg F.L., Rifkin M.D., Ultrasound examination of the hand. Radiology 1985, 155: 785–788

Fornage B.D., Soft-tissue changes in the hand in rheumatoid arthritis: evaluation with US. Radiology 1989, 173: 735–737

Gooding G.A.W., Tenosynovitis of the wrist: a sonographic demonstration. J Ultrasound Med 1988, 7: 225–226

Hentz V.R., Green P.S., Arditi M., Imaging studies of the cadaver hand using transmission ultrasound. Skeletal Radiol 1987, 16: 474–480

Hentz V.R., Marich K.W., Parvati Dev Ph. D., Preliminary study of the upper limb with the use ultrasound transmission imaging. J Hand Surg 1984, 9-A: 188–193

Hergan K., Mittler C., Oser W., Ulnar collateral ligament: differentiation of displaced and nondisplaced tears with US and MR imaging. Radiology 1995, 194: 65–71

Mannerfelt L., Norman O., Attrition ruptures of flexor tendons in rheumatoid arthritis caused by bony spurs in the carpal tunnel. J Bone Joint Surg 1969, 51-B: 270–277

McGeorge D.D., McGeorge S., Diagnostic medical ultrasound in the management of hand injuries. J Hand Surg 1990, 15-B: 256–261

Nelson C.L., Sawmiller S., Phalen G.S., Ganglions of the wrist and hand. J Bone Joint Surg 1972, 54-A: 1459–1464

Noszian I.M., Dinkhauser L.M., Orthner E., Straub G.M., Csanady M., Ulnar collateral ligament: differentiation of displaced and nondisplaced tears with US. Radiology 1995, 194: 61–63

O'Callaghan B.I., Kohut G., Hoogewoud H.M., Gamekeeper thumb: identification of the Stener lesion with US. Radiology 1994, 192: 477–480

Schernberg F., Fornage B., Collin J.P., Ameil M., Sandre J., L'échographie en temps réel: une méthode d'imagerie de la main. Ann Chir Main 1987, 6: 239–244

Seboun P., Souissi M., Ebelin M., Rigot J., Dabos N., Moreau J.F., Exploration ultrasonographique des parties molles de la main: Tumeurs et pseudo-tumeurs des parties molles. Résultats préliminaires à propos de 12 cas opérés. J Radiol 1989, 70: 346–351

Souissi M., Ebelin M., Rigot J., Lemerle J.P., Moreau J.F., Exploration ultrasonographique des parties molles de la main: Pathologie traumatique et inflammatoire des tendons fléchisseurs des doigts de la main. J Radiol 1989, 70: 352–355

Souissi M., Giwerc M., Ebelin M., Richard O., Cyna-Gorse F., Moreau J.F., Exploration ultrasonographique des parties molles de la main: Technique d'examen et anatomie normale de la paume de la main. J Radiol 1989, 70: 337–345

Souissi M., Giwerc M., Ebelin M., Rigot J., Richard O., Seboun Ph., Lemerle J.P., Moreau J.F., Exploration échographique des tendons fléchisseurs des doigts de la main. Presse Med 1989, 18: 463–466

Sullivan P.P., Berquist T.H., Magnetic resonance imaging of the hand, wirst, and forearm: utility in patients with pain and dysfunction as a result of trauma. Mayo Clin Proc 1991, 66: 1217–1221

Weiss K.L., Beltran J., Lubbers L.M., High-field MR surface-coil imaging of the hand and wrist: pathologic correlations and clinical relevance. Radiology 1986, 160: 147–152

Weiss K.L., Beltran J., Shamam O.M., Stilla R.F., Levey M.: High-field MR surface-coil imaging of the hand and wrist: normal anatomy. Radiology 1986, 160: 143–146

Pediatric Hip

Adam R., Hendry G.M.A., Moss J., Wild S.R., Gillespie I., Arthrosonography of the irritable hip in childhood: a review of 1 year's experience. Br J Radiol 1986, 59: 205–208

Alexander J.E., Seibert J.J., Glasier C.M., Williamson S.L., Aronson J., McCarthy R.E., Rodgers A.B., Corbitt S.L., High-resolution hip ultrasound in the limping child. J Clin Ultrasound 1989, 17: 19–24

Berman L., Catterall A., Meire H.B., Ultrasound of the hip: a review of the application of a new technique. Br J Radiol 1986, 59: 13–17

Berman L., Klenerman L., Ultrasound screening for hip abnormalities: preliminary findings in 1001 neonates. Br Med J 1986, 293: 719–722

Bickerstaff D.R., Neal L.M., Booth A.J., Brennan P.O., Bell M.J., Ultrasound examination of the irritable hip. J Bone Joint Surg 1990, 72-B: 549–553

Boal D.K.B., Schwenkter E.P., The enfant hip: assessment with real-time US. Radiology 1985, 157: 667–672

Castriota-Scanderbeg A., De Micheli V., Orsi E., Ultrasound and hip joint effusion. Eur J Radiol 1993, 17: 133–134

Castriota-Scanderbeg A., De Micheli V., Orsi E., Ultrasound and hip joint effusion. Eur J Radiol 1994, 18: 74–75

Cheng I.H., Kuo K.N., Lubicky J.P., Prognosticating factors in acetabular development following reduction of developmental dysplasia of the hip. J Pediatr Orthop 1994, 14: 3–8

Cheng J.C.Y., Chan Y.L., Hui P.W., Shen W.Y., Metreweli C., Ultrasonographic hip morphometry in infants. J Pediatr Orthop 1994, 14: 24–28

Clarke N.M.P., Clegg J., Al-Chalabi A.N., Ultrasound screening of hips at risk for CDH. J Bone Joint Surg 1989, 71-B: 9–12

Clarke N.M.P., Harcke H.T., McHugh P., Lee M.S., Borns P.F., MacEwen G.D., Real-time ultrasound in the diagnosis of congenital dislocation and dysplasia of the hip. J Bone Joint Surg 1985, 67-B: 406–412

Dahlström H., Oberg L., Friberg S., Sonography in congenital dislocation of the hip. Acta Orthop Scand 1986, 57: 402–406

Egund N., Wingstrand H., Forsberg L., Pettersson H., Sundén G., Computed tomography and ultrasonography for diagnosis of hip joint effusion in children. Acta Orthop Scand 1986, 57: 211–215

Gerscovich E.O., Greenspan A., Cronan M.S., Karol L.A., McGahan J.P., Three-dimensional sonographic evaluation of developmental dysplasia of the hip: preliminary findings. Radiology 1994, 190: 407–410

Gomes H., Menanteau B., Motte J., Robiliard P., Sonography of the neonatal hip: a dynamic approach. Ann Radiol 1987, 30: 503–510

Graf R., Classification of hip joint dysplasia by means of sonography. Arch Orthop Trauma Surg 1984, 102: 248–255

Graf R., The diagnosis of congenital hip-joint dislocation by the ultrasonic combound treatment. Arch Orthop Traumat Surg 1980, 97: 117–133

Grissom L.E., Harcke H.T., Kumar S.J., Bassett G.S., MacEwen G.D., Ultrasound evaluation of hip position in the Pavlik harness. J Ultrasound Med 1988, 7: 1–6

Grissom L.E., Harcke H.T., Sonography in congenital deficiency of the femur. J Pediatr Orthop 1994, 14: 29–33

Harcke H.T., Clarke N.M.P., Lee M.S., Borns P.F., MacEwen G.D., Examination of the infant hip with real-time ultrasonography. J Ultrasound Med 1984, 3: 131–137

Harcke H.T., Grissom L.E., Performing dynamic sonography of the infant hip. AJR 1990, 155: 837–844

Harcke H.T., Lee M.S., Sinning L., Clarke N.M.P., Borns P.F., MacEwen G.D., Ossification Center of the infant hip: sonographic and radiographic correlation. AJR 1986, 147: 317–321

Hinderaker T., Uden A., Reikeras O., Direct ultrasonographic measurement of femoral anterversion in newborns. Skeletal Radiol 1994, 23: 133–135

References

Kallio P., Ryöppy S., Jäppinen S., Siponmaa A.K., Jääskeläinen J., Kunnamo I., Ultrasonography in hip disease in children. Acta Orthop Scand 1985, 56: 367–371

Keller M.S., Chawla H.S., Sonographic delineation of the neonatal acetabular labrum. J Ultrasound Med 1985, 4: 501–502

Keller M.S., Weltin G.G., Rattner Z., Taylor K.J.W., Rosenfield N.S., Normal instability of the hip in the neonate. Radiology 1988, 169: 733–736

Krasny R., Prescher A., Botschek A., Lemke R., Casser H.R., Adam G., MR-anatomy of infants hip: comparison to anatomical preparations. Pediatr Radiol 1991, 21: 211–215

Kumasaka Y., Harada K., Watanabe H., Higashihara T., Kishimoto H., Sakurai K., Kozuka T., Modified epiphyseal index for MRI in Legg-Calve-Perthes disease. Pediatr Radiol 1991, 21: 208–210

Langer R., Ultrasonic investigation of the hip in newborns in the diagnosis of congenital hip dislocation: classification and results of a screening program. Skeletal Radiol 1987, 16: 275–279

Marchal G.J., van Holsbeeck M.T., Raes M., Favril A.A., Verbeken E.E., Casteels Vandaele M., Baert A.L., Lauweryns J.M., Transient synovitis of the hip in children: role of US. Radiology 1987, 162: 825–828

Markowitz R.I., Davidson R.S., Harty M.P., Bellah R.D., Hubbard A.M., Rosenberg H.K., Sonography of the elbow in infants and children. AJR 1992, 159: 829–833

Miralles M., Gonzales G., Pulpeiro J.R., Millan J.M., Gordillo I., Serrano C., Olcoz F., Martinez A., Sonography of the painful hip in children: 500 consecutive cases. AJR 1989, 152: 579–582

Morin C., Harcke H.T., MacEwen G.D., The infant hip: real-time US assessment of acetabular development. Radiology 1985, 157: 673–677

Novick G., Ghelman B., Schneider M., Sonography of the neonatal and infant hip. AJR 1983, 141: 639–645

Novick G.S., Sonography in pediatric hip disorders. Radiol Clin North Am 1988, 26: 29–53

O'Sullivan M.E., O'Brien T., Acetabular dysplasia presenting as developmental dislocation of the hip. J Pediatr Orthop 1994, 14: 13–15

Schlesinger A.E., Hernandez R.J., Diseases of the musculoskeletal system in children: imaging with CT, sonography, and MR. AJR 1992, 158: 729–741

Scott S.T., Infant hip ultrasound. Clin Radiol 1989, 40: 551–553

Sellier N., Koifman P., Demange Ph., Kalifa G., Echographie de la hanche du nourisson. Ann Radiol 1993, 36: 22–26

Soboleski D.A., Babyn P., Sonographic diagnosis of developmental dysplasia of the hip: importance of increased thickness of acetabular cartilage. AJR 1993, 161: 839–842

Suzuki S., Awaya G., Okada Y., Ikeda T., Tada H., Examination by ultrasound of Legg-Calvé-Perthes disease. Clin Orthop 1987, 220: 130–135

Tanaka T., Yoshihashi Y., Miura T., Changes in soft tissue interposition after reduction of developmental dislocation of the hip. J Pediatr Orthop 1994, 14: 16–23

Terjesen T., Osthus P., Ultrasound in the diagnosis and follow-up of transient synovitis of the hip. J Pediatr Orthop 1991, 11: 608–613

Terjesen T., Ultrasonography in the primary evaluation of patients with Perthes disease. J Pediatr Orthop 1993, 13: 437–443

Wingstrand H., Egund N., Ultrasonography in hip joint effusion. Acta Orthop Scand 1984, 55: 469–471

Hip

Berman L., Catterall A., Meire H.B., Ultrasound of the hip: a review of the applications of a new technique. Br J Radiol 1986, 59: 13–17

Claudon M., Regent D., Tonnel F., Donze F., Fery A., Tréheux A., La trochantérite tuberculeuse: intérêt de l'échographie et de la scanographie. J Radiol 1986, 67: 309–314

Földes K., Gaal M., Balint P., Nemenyi K., Kiss C., Balint G.P., Buchanan W.W., Ultrasonography after hip arthroplasty. Skeletal Radiol 1992, 21: 297–299

Gerscovich E.O., Greenspan A., Cronan M.S., Karol L.A., McGahan J.P., Three-dimensional sonographic evaluation of developmental dysplasia of the hip: preliminary findings. Radiology 1994, 190: 407–410

Gitschlag K.F., Sandler M.A., Madrazo B.L., Hricak H., Eyler W.R., Disease in the femoral triangle: sonographic appearance. AJR 1982, 139: 515–519

Graif M., Strauss S., Heim M., Itzchak Y., Sonography of the hip joint as part of the evaluation of acute lower abdominal pain. J Clin Ultrasound 1988, 16: 99–102

Komppa G.H., Northern J.R., Haas D.K., Lisecki E., Ghaed N., Ultrasound guidance for needle aspiration of the hip in patients with painful hip prosthesis. J Clin Ultrasound 1985, 13: 433–434

Linder L., Lindberg L., Carlsson A., Aseptic loosening of hip prostheses. Clin Orthop 1983, 175: 93–104

Moulton A., Upadhyay S.S., A direct method of measuring femoral anteversion using ultrasound. J Bone Joint Surg 1982, 64-B: 469–472

O'Sullivan M.E., O'Brien T., Acetabular dysplasia presenting as developmental dislocation of the hip. J Pediatr Orthop 1994, 14: 13–15

Solobeski D.A., Babyn P., Sonographic diagnosis of developmental dysplasia of the hip: importance of increased thickness of acetabular cartilage. AJR 1993, 161: 839–842

Staple T.W., Arthrographic demonstration of iliopsoas bursa extension of the hip joint. Radiology 1972, 102: 515–516

Upadhyay S.S., O'Neil T., Burwell R.G., Moulton A., A new method using ultrasound for measuring femoral anteversion (torsion): technique and reliability. Br J Radiol 1987, 60: 519–523

van Holsbeeck M.T., Eyler W.R., Sherman L.S., Lombardi T.J., Mezger E., Verner J.J., Schurman J.R., Jonsson K., Detection of infection in loosened hip prostheses: efficacy of sonography. AJR 1994, 163: 381–384

Wilson D.J., Green D.J., McLarnon J.C., Arthrosonography of the painful hip. Clin Radiol 1984, 35: 17–19

Wilson P.D., Salvati E.A., Aglietti P., Kutner L.J., The problem of infection in endoprosthetic surgery of the hip joint. Clin Orthop 1973, 96: 213–221

Zarate R., Cuny C., Sazos P., Détermination de l'antéversion du col du fémur par échographie. J Radiol 1983, 64: 307–311

Knee

Aisen A.M., McCune W.J., MacGuire A., Carson P.L., Silver T.M., Jafri S.Z., Martel W., Sonographic evaluation of the cartilage of the knee. Radiology 1984, 153: 781–784

Ambanelli U., Manganelli P., Nervetti A., Ugolotti U., Demonstration of articular effusions and popliteal cysts with ultrasound. J Rheumatol 1976, 3: 134–139

Armstrong S.J., Watt I., Lipoma arborescens of the knee. Br J Radiol 1989, 62: 178–180

Barrie H.J., The pathogenesis and significance of meniscal cysts. J Bone Joint Surg 1979, 61-B: 184–189

Corbetti F., Schiavon F., Fiocco U., Angelini F., Gambari P.F., Unusual antefemoral dissecting cyst. Br J Radiol 1985, 58: 675–677

De Flaviis L., Nessi R., Scaglione P., Balconi G., Albisetti W., Derchi L.E., Ultrasonic diagnosis of Osgood-Schlatter and Sinding-Larsen-Johansson diseases of the knee. Skeletal Radiol 1989, 18: 193–197

Derks W.H.J., de Hooge P., van Linge B., Ultrasonographic detection of the patellar plica in the knee. J Clin Ultrasound 1986, 14: 355–360

Fornage B.D., Rifkin M.D., Touche D.H., Segal Ph.M., Sonography of the patellar tendon: preliminary observations. AJR 1984, 143: 179–182

Fornage B.D., Touche D., Deshayes J.L., Segal Ph., Diagnostic des calcifications du tendon rotulien: comparaison écho-radiographique. J Radiol 1984, 65: 355–359

Frank C., Amiel D., Akeson W.H., Healing of the medial collateral ligament of the knee. Acta Orthop Scand 1983, 54: 917–923

Gagnerie F., Taillan B., Bruneton J.N., Bonnard J.M., Denis F., Commandre F., Euller-Ziegler L., Ziegler G., Three cases of pigmented villonodular synovitis of the knee. Fortschr Röntgenstr 1986, 145: 227–228

Gompels B.M., Darlington L.G., Evaluation of popliteal cysts and painful calves with ultrasonography: comparison with arthrography. Ann Rheum Dis 1982, 41: 355–359

Gordon G.V., Edell S., Brogadir S.P., Schumacher H.R., Schimmer B.M.,Dalinka M., Baker's cysts and true thrombophlebitis. Arch Intern Med 1979, 139: 40–42

Gordon G.V., Edell S., Ultrasonic evaluation of popliteal cysts. Arch Intern Med 1980, 140: 1453–1455

Hall F.M., Joffe N., CT Imaging of the anserine bursa. AJR 1988, 150: 1107–1108

Hastings D.E., Knee ligament instability-a rational anatomical classification. Clin Orthop 1986, 208: 104–107

Hastings D.E., The non-operative management of collateral ligament injuries of the knee joint. Clin Orthop 1980, 147: 22–28

Hermann G., Yeh H.C., Lehr-Janus C., Berson B.L., Diagnosis of popliteal cyst: double-contrast arthrography and sonography. AJR 1981, 137: 369–372

Ismail A.M., Balakrishnan R., Rajakumar M.K., Rupture of patellar ligament after steroid infiltration. J Bone Joint Surg 1969, 51-B: 503–505

Kälebo P., Swärd L., Karlsson J., Peterson L., Ultrasonography in the detection of partial patellar ligament ruptures-jumper's knee. Skeletal Radiol 1991, 20: 285–289

Kelly D.W., Carter V.S., Jobe F.W., Kerlan R.K., Patellar and quadriceps tendon ruptures-jumper's knee. Am J Sports Med 1984, 12: 375–380

King J.B., Perry D.J., Mourad K., Kumar S.J., Lesions of the patellar ligament. J Bone Joint Surg 1990, 72-B: 46–48

Kricun R., Kricun M.E., Arangio G.A., Salzman G.S., Berman A.T., Patellar tendon rupture with underlying systemic disease. AJR 1980, 135: 803–807

Laine H.R., Harjula A., Peltokallio P. , Ultrasound in the evaluation of the knee and patellar regions. J Ultrasound Med 1987, 6: 33–36

Lanning P., Heikkinen E., Ultrasonic features of the Osgood-Schlatter lesion. J Pediatr Orthop 1991, 11: 538–540

Lindgren P.G., Willén R., Gastrocnemio-semimembranosus bursa and its relation to the knee joint. Acta Radiol Diagn 1977, 18: 497–512

Lukes P.J., Herberts P., Zachrisson B.E., Ultrasound in the diagnosis of popliteal cysts. Acta Radiol Diagn 1980, 21: 663–665

Martino F., Ettorre G.C., Angelelli G., Macarini L., Patella V., Moretti B., D'Amore M., Cantatore F.P., Validity of echographic evaluation of cartilage in gonarthrosis. Preliminary report. Clin Rheumatol 1993, 12:178–183

McDonald D.G., Leopold G.R., Ultrasound B-scanning in the differentiation of Baker's cyst and thrombophlebitis. Br J Radiol 1972, 45: 729–732

Meehan P.L., Daftari T., Pigmented villonodular synovitis presenting as a popliteal cyst in a child. J Bone Joint Surg 1994, 76-A: 593–595

Moore C.P., Sarti D.A., Louie J.S., Ultrasonographic demonstration of popliteal cysts in rheumatoid arthritis. Arthritis Rheum 1975, 18: 577–580

Mourad K., King J., Guggiana P., Computed tomography and ultrasound imaging of jumper's knee – patellar tendinitis. Clin Radiol 1988, 39: 162–165

Myllysmäki T., Bondestam S., Suramo I., Cederberg A., Peltokallio P., Ultrasonography of jumper's knee. Acta Radiol 1990, 31: 147–149

Noble C.A., Iliotibial band friction syndrome in runners. Am J Sports Med 1980, 8: 232–234

Pathria M.N., Zlatkin M., Sartoris D.J., Scheible W., Resnick D., Ultrasonography of the popliteal fossa and lower extremities. Radiol Clin North Am 1988, 26: 77–85

Peetrons P., Allaer D., Jeanmart L., Cysts of the semilunar cartilages of the knee: a new approach by ultrasound imaging. J Ultrasound Med 1990, 9: 333–337

Reuter K.L., Raptopoulos V., DeGiromali U., Akins C.M., Ultrasonography of a plexiform neurofibroma of the popliteal fossa. J Ultrasound Med 1982, 1: 209–211

Richardson M.L., Selby B., Montana M.A., Mack L.A., Ultrasonography of the knee. Radiol Clin North Am 1988, 26: 63–75

Schwimmer M., Edelstein G., Heiken J.P., Gilula L.A., Synovial cysts of the knee: CT Evaluation. Radiology 1985, 154: 175–177

Selby B., Richardson M.L., Nelson B.D., Graney D.O., Mack L.A., Sonography in the detection of meniscal injuries of the knee: evaluation in cadavers. AJR 1987, 149: 549–553

Stern R.E., Harwin S.F., Spontaneous and simultaneous rupture of both quadriceps tendons. Clin Orthop 1980, 147: 188–189

Strejcek J., Popelka S., Bilateral rupture of the patellar ligaments in systemic lupus erythematosus. Lancet 1969: 743

Teitz C.C., Ultrasonography in the knee: clinical aspects. Radiol Clin North Am 1988, 26: 55–62

Toolanen G., Lorentzon R., Friberg S., Dahlström H., Oberg L., Sonography of popliteal masses. Acta Orthop Scand 1988, 59: 294–296

Vahey T.N., Broome D.R., Kayes K.J., Shelbourne K.D., Acute and chronic tears of the anterior cruciate ligament: differential features at MR imaging. Radiology 1991, 181: 251–253

van Holsbeeck M., van Holsbeeck K., Gevers G., Marchal G., van Steen A., Favril A., Gielen J., Dequeker J., Baert A., Staging and follow-up of rheumatoid arthritis of the knee: comparison of sonography, thermography, and clinical assessment. J Ultrasound Med 1988, 7: 561–566

References

Ankle and foot

Aström M., Westlin N., Blood flow in chronic Achilles tendinopathy. Clin Orthop 1994, 308: 166–172

Bianchi S., Zwass A., Abdelwahab I.F., Zoccola C., Evaluation of tibialis anterior tendon rupture by ultrasonography. J Clin Ultrasound 1994, 22: 564–566

Blei C.L., Nirschl R.P., Grant E.G., Achilles tendon: US diagnosis of pathologic conditions. Radiology 1986, 159: 765–767

Canta-Melian B., Assiaza-Loureda R., Aisa-Vasela P., Tibialis posterior nerve schwannoma mimicking Achilles tendinitis ultrasonographic diagnosis. J Clin Ultrasound 1990, 18: 671–673

Church C.C., Radiographic diagnosis of acute peroneal tendon dislocation. AJR 1977, 129: 1065–1068

Downey D.J., Simkin P.A., Mack L.A., Richardson M.L., Kilcoyne R.F., Hansen S.T., Tibialis posterior tendon rupture: a cause of rheumatoid flat foot. Arthritis Rheum 1988, 31: 441–446

Ekstrom J.E., Shuman W.P., Mack L.A., MR imaging of accessory soleus muscle. J. Comp Assist Tomogr 1990, 14: 239–242

Fornage B.D., Achilles tendon: US examination. Radiology 1986, 159: 759–764

Fornage B.D., Richli W.R., Chuapetcharasopon Ch., Calcaneal bone cyst: sonographic findings and ultrasound-guided aspiration biopsy. J Clin Ultrasound 1991, 19: 360–362

Fornage B.D., Rifkin M.D., Ultrasound examination of the hand and foot. Radiol Clin North Am 1988, 26: 109–129

Friedrich J.M., Schnarkowski P., Rübenacker S., Wallner B., Ultrasonography of capsular morphology in normal and traumatic ankle joints. J Clin Ultrasound 1993, 21: 179–187

Funk D.A., Cass J.R., Johnson K.A., Acquired adult flat foot secondary to posterior tibial-tendon pathology. J Bone Joint Surg 1986, 68-A: 95–102

Gooding G.A.W., Stess R.M., Graf P.M., Moss K.M., Louie K.S., Grunfeld C., Sonography of the sole of the foot: evidence for loss of foot pad thickness in diabetes and its relationship to ulceration of the foot. Invest Radiol 1986, 21: 45–48

Gooding G.A.W., Stress R.M., Graf P.M., Grunfeld C., Heel pad thickness: determination by high-resolution ultrasonography. J Ultrasound Med 1985, 4: 173–174

Inglis A.E., Scott W.N., Sculco T.P., Patterson A.H., Ruptures of the tendo Achillis. J. Bone Joint Surg 1976, 58-A: 990–993

Kainberger F.M., Engel A., Barton P., Huebsch P., Neuhold A., Salomonowitz E., Injury of the Achilles tendon: diagnosis with sonography. AJR 1990, 155: 1031–1036

Karasick D., Schweitzer M.E., Tear of the posterior tibial tendon causing asymmetric flat foot: radiologic findings. AJR 1993, 161: 1237–1240

Laine H.R., Harjula A.L.J., Peltokallio P., Ultrasonography as a differential diagnostic aid in achillodynia. J Ultrasound Med 1987, 6: 351–362

Leekam R.N., Salsberg B.B, Bogoch E., Shankar L., Sonographic diagnosis of partial Achilles tendon rupture and healing. J Ultrasound Med 1986, 5: 115–116

Mann R.A., Thompson F.M., Rupture of posterior tibial tendon causing flat foot. J Bone Joint Surg 1985, 67-A: 556–561

Mathieson J.R., Connell D.G., Cooperberg P.L., Lloyd-Smith D.R., Sonography of the Achilles tendon and adjacent bursae. AJR 1988, 151: 127–131

McConkey J.P., Favero K.J., Subluxation of the peroneal tendons within the peroneal tendon sheath: a case report. Am J Sports Med 1987, 15: 511–513

Morrison W.B., Schweitzer M.E., Wapner K.L., Lackman R.D., Plantar fibromatosis: a benign aggressive neoplasm with a characteristic appearance on MR images. Radiology 1994, 193: 841–845

Redd R.A., Peter V.J., Emery S.F., Branch H.M., Rifkin M.D., Morton neuroma sonographic evaluation. Radiology 1989, 171: 415–417

Reed M., Gooding G.A.W., Kerley S.M., Himebaugh M.S., Griswold V.J., Sonography of plantar fibromatosis. J Clin Ultrasound 1991, 19: 578–582

Steinmetz A., Schmitt W., Schuler P., Kleinsorge F., Schneider J., Kaffarnik H., Ultrasonography of Achilles tendons in primary hypercholesterolemia: comparison with computed tomography. Atherosclerosis 1988, 74: 231–239

Stephenson C.A., Seibert J.J., McAndrew M.P., Glasier C.M., Leithiser R.E., Iqbal V., Sonographic diagnosis of tenosynovitis of the posterior tibial tendon. J Clin Ultrasound 1990, 18: 114–116

Taziaux B., Morice J.E., Echographie du pied et de la cheville. Sauramps Medical 1994

Vazelle F., Rochcongar P., Masse M., Ramée A., La pathologie du tendon d'Achille. J Radiol 1981, 62: 299–307

Yu J.S., Witte D., Resnick D., Pogue W., Ossification of the Achilles tendon: imaging abnormalities in 12 patients. Skeletal Radiol 1994, 23: 127–131

Yuzawa K., Yamakawa K., Tohno E., Seki M., Akisada M., Yanagi H., Okafuji T., Yamanouchi Y., Hattori N., Kawai K., Shimakura Y., Tsuchiya S., Ijima H., Fukao K., Wasaki Y., Hamaguchi H., An ultrasonographic method for detection of Achilles tendon xanthomas in familial hypercholesterolemia. Atherosclerosis 1989, 75: 211–218

Index

A

acetabulum, anatomy 122–125
  infant hip, anatomy 118, 120
Achilles tendon, *see* tendon
acromion, anatomy 63
  impingement syndrome 70
algoneurodystrophia 53
amyloid, subscapular tendon 32
  wrist 106
ankle, *see* tendon Achilles
ankle, bursitis 171
  Haglund deformity 174
  joint loose body 162
    effusion 162
  ligament injury 172
  peroneal synovitis 167
    tendon luxation 168
  posterior tibial tendon, rupture 170
    tenosynovitis 169
  tenosynovial cyst 175
aponeurosis, palmar, anatomy 110, 179,
    180
  plantar, fasciitis 185
    Ledderhose disease 186
    rupture 185
artery, anterior tibial, anatomy 158
  brachial, anatomy 17, 77, 78, 80
  circumflex, lateral femoral, anatomy
    122
    medial femoral anatomy 125
  common femoral, pseudoaneurysm 43
  popliteal, aneurysm 43
    calcifications 43
  radial, anatomy 92, 93, 96
  ulnar, anatomy 91, 92, 94
arthritis, rheumatoid, Achilles tendon
    165
  ankle 162, 171
  bursitis 37
  elbow 88, 89
  foot 181
  hand 112
  hip 126
  knee 58
  synovial thickening 41
  tendinitis 32
  wrist 103
  septic 39, 40
    hip 126
    puncture 58
  wrist 100
arthroscopy, knee 144
artifacts, absent shadow 6
  acoustic shadow 24, 25, 40, 64, 71,
    86, 129, 185
  anisotropy 8,18
  beamwidth 6
  calcifications 6
  comet's tail 10, 57
  critical angle shadowing 9
  dirty shadow 10
  enhancement, by transmission 7
    posterior 7
  refractile shadowing 6,9
  repetitive echogenic bands 10

reverberation 10
  tendon 8
    Achillles 9
  time gain compensation 7
aspiration, septic arthritis 40

B

Baker's cyst, *see* cyst
band, iliotibial, shin splint 150
bell-clapper sign 22
bone, anatomy 14
  cortex, fracture 47
    osteomyelitis 49
    stress fracture 48
  cuboid, anatomy 176
  cuneiform, anatomy 177, 179
  foot, injury 184
  fracture, callus formation 48, 50
  metacarpal, anatomy 109
    Dupuytren's contracture 114
  metatarsal, anatomy 176–179
    fracture 184
    gout 182
  osteomyelitis, acute 49
    chronic 49, 52
      MRI 49
  periosteum, fracture 47
    infection 50
    osteomyelitis 49
    periosteal desmoid 154
    stress fracture 48
  subchondral, degeneration 42
bursa, anatomy 15
  foot 183
  foreign body 37
  gastrocnemius-semimembranosus,
    anatomy 15
    synovial thickening 37
  iliopsoasbursitis 128
  inferior patellar bursitis, acute 38
  infrapatellar bursitis 148
  olecranon bursitis 37, 89
  prepatellar bursitis 37, 148
    acute 36
  retrocalcaneal, anatomy 157
    bursitis 171, 174
  subacromial, impingement syndrome
    69
  subacromial-subdeltoid, anatomy 15
    bursitis 69–70
    effusion 69
    Geiser sign 67
    rotator cuff full-thickness tear 65,
      66
  subdeltoid, anatomy 60–62
    bursitis, calcifications 71
      hemorrhagic 38
    Milwaukee shoulder 75
    rotator cuff full-thickness tear 66
  suprapatellar, anatomy 15
  trochanteric, bursitis 128
bursitis, acute 36
  ankle, bursitis 171
  chronic 36, 38

de novo 36
foot 183
frictional 36, 38
hemorrhagic 38
infectious 37
inflammatory 37
metabolic 38
pes anserinus tendinitis 147
plantar fasciitis 185
puncture 58
septic 37
traumatic 38

C

calcaneum, accessory soleus muscle 173
  anatomy 157, 160, 177–180
  fracture, peroneal tendon injury 167
  plantar fasciitis 185
  retrocalcaneal bursitis 171
canal, Guyon's 104
capitulum, anatomy 79–82
capsule, effusion 39
  effusion, septic 40
  loose bodies 40, 42
  synovial thickening 41
carpal tunnel syndrome, *see* nerve,
    median
carpal tunnel syndrome 45
carpe bossu 99
cartilage, articular, ulcerations 42
  elbow, anatomy 80
  fibrocartilage, anatomy 16
  fragments 40
  hyaline, anatomy 16, 109
    foot 176
    humeral head 61
    infant hip 119
    talar 158, 159
    fracture 42
  interface sign 65
  trauma 42
  triradiate, infant hip, anatomy 119,
    120
chondromalacia 39
clavicle, anatomy 63
compartment syndrome 27
condyle, femoral, lateral, shin splint
    150
    medial, degeneration 42
    periosteal desmoid 154
contracture, *see* Dupuytren
cortex, metatarsal fracture 184
corticoid injection 40
cyst, arthrosynovial, elbow 88
  foot 183
  wrist 97
  Baker's 36, 37, 40
  epidermoid, sebaceous 55
  foot 183
  ganglion cyst, ankle 175
    knee 153
    wrist 98
  meniscal 152
  metatarsophalangeal 183

Index

cyst *(cont.)*
  muscular 25
  pisiform 104
  radiolunate 97
  radioscaphoid 97
  scaphotrapezoid 97
  subcutaneous 55
  synovial, wrist 99
  tenosynovial, ankle 175
    hand 115

D

De Quervain's tenosynovitis 101
desmoid, periosteal, knee 154
diabetes, Achilles tendon rupture 165
diffuse idiopathic skeletal hyperostosis
  (DISH),174
Dupuytren's contracture 114

E

elbow, bursitis, frictional 85
  epicondylitis 86
  golfer's 86
  rheumatoid arthritis 89
  tennis 86
eminence, hypothenar, anatomy 110
  thenar, anatomy 107
entesopathy, ankle 174
entesophyte, olecranon 87
  plantar fasciitis 185
enthesis trauma, hip 130
epicondyle, anatomy 80
  lateral, anatomy 81
  medial, anatomy 81–83, 86
    lipoma 54
    ulnar nerve entrapment 88
epicondylitis, lateral 86
equipment, high frequency transducer
  19
  linear array probe 3
  transducer 2
erysipelas 44, 53
examination technique 3
  compression 4,17
  contraction 5
  dynamic 12
  high frequency transducer 19
  tendon, contralateral 12
  testing maneuvers, ankle 158

F

fascia, plantar, fasciitis 185
fat, anatomy 19
  Hoffa 144
    Osgood-Schlatter disease 145
  Kager's, Achilles tendon tendinitis
    163
  subcutaneous, anatomy 19
  knee, fluid collection 149
femur, anatomy 122, 125
  condyle, medial, degeneration 42
    synovial impingement 147
  infant hip, anatomy 118
  periosteal desmoid 154
fibrocartilage, anatomy 16
  triangular, anatomy 94

cleft 105
fibromatosis, plantar 186
fibula, anatomy 155, 156, 158, 159
  fracture 47
  malleolus, anatomy 160
finger, *see* Mallet finger
flexor retinacaculum, carpal tunnel
  syndrome 104
foot, bone injury 184
  cystic mass 183
  Ledderhose disease 186
  Morton neuroma 183, 187
  plantar fasciitis 185
foreign body 56, 57
  glass 57
  plastic 57
fossa, coronoid, anatomy 79
  loose bodies 84
  olecranon, anatomy 81, 82, 83
    effusion 84
    hemarthrosis 84
fracture, calcaneum, peroneal tendon
  injury 167
  stress 45

G

gamekeeper's thumb 116
ganglion cyst, ankle 175
  knee 153
    MRI 153
  pathogensis 98
  wrist 98
Geiser sign 67
glass, *see* foreign body
golfer's elbow 86
gout, ankle 165
  bursitis 38
  elbow 85
  foot 182
  knee 148
  tendinitis 32
  wrist 100, 104
groove, biceps tendon 62
  bicipital, degeneration 72
    effusion 74
    empty 73
  condylar, anatomy 16
Guyon, canal syndrome 104

H

Haglund deformity, ankle 174
hallux, valgus 183
hand, Dupuytren's contracture 114
  gamekeeper's thumb 116
  osteoarthritis 114
  rheumatoid arthritis 112
  tendon, rupture 113
    tenosynovitis 112
  tenosynovial cyst 115
hemarthrosis 39
  elbow 84
hemodialysis 32, 38, 106
Hill–Sachs lesion 47, 76
hip, bursitis 128
  effusion 126
    septic 40
  enthesis trauma 130
  hydroxyapatite cristal deposit 129

infant, anatomy 118–121
  effusion 127
  synovitis 127
Legg–Calve–Perthes disease 127
rheumatoid arthritis 126
sports injury 130
tendinitis 129
Hoffa's fat see fat
humerus, *see* Hill–Sachs lesion
  anatomy 16, 78
  lesser tuberosity, anatomy 64
    biceps tendon luxation 73
  Milwaukee shoulder 75
hydroxyapatite cristal deposit, hip 129
hypothenar, *see* muscle

I

Ilizarov procedure 50
impingement, syndrome 67, 69, 70
  synovial, knee 147
infant hip, anatomy 119
injury, cruciate ligament 151
  knee 149
  plantar aponeurosis 185
  sports, knee 149
ischium, anatomy 123

J

joint capsule see capsule
joint coxofemoral, *see* hip
joint, acromioclavicular, anatomy 63
  luxation 76
    sprain 76
  ankle, rheumatoid arthritis 162
  arthrosynovial cyst 183
  capsule, anatomy 15
    coxofemoral, anatomy 15
  carpometacarpal, degenerative 114
  fibulotalar, anatomy 159
  glenohumeral, anatomy 62
    destruction 75
    effusion 74
  interphalangeal, rheumatoid arthritis
    112
  lunocapitate, rheumatoid arthritis
    103
  metacarpo-phalangeal, foreign body
    56
    anatomy 108, 109
    rheumatoid arthritis 112
  metatarsal-phalangeal, anatomy 176
    gout 182
    rheumatoid arthritis 181
  midtarsal, posterior tibial tendon
    rupture 170
  radiocarpal, synovial thickening 41
  radiohumeral, anatomy 79
  radiolunate, rheumatoid arthritis 103
  radioscaphoid, rheumatoid arthritis
    103
  subtalar, loose bodies 40
  talonavicular, rheumatoid arthritis
    181
  tarsal, rheumatoid arthritis 181
  tibiotalar, anatomy 158
jumper's knee 3, 143

K

Kager's triangle, anatomy 157, 161
  cystic mass 175
  accessory soleus muscle 173
knee, arthroscopy 144
  bursitis 148
  calcification 144
  calcified enthesopathy 146
  cruciate ligament, injury 151
  entheses, ossification 144
  epycondyle, lateral, foreign body 57
  ganglion cyst 153
  injury 149
  jumper's knee 3
  meniscal tear 152
  meniscus, internal, anatomy 16
    injury 42
  Osgood-Schlatter disease 145
  patellar tendinitis, chronic 144
  periosteal desmoid 154
  pes anserinus tendinitis 147
  retinaculum, synovial impingement
    147
  runner's knee 150
  shin splint 150
  Stieda-Pellegrini syndrome 149
  total prosthesis 51
  valgus stress 149, 152
  varus stress 152

L

labrum, anatomy 122, 125
  infant hip 119
Ledderhose disease 186
Legg-Calve-Perthes disease 127
ligament, anatomy 13
  ankle, injury 172
  annular, anatomy 79, 176
  anterior, cruciate, rupture 149, 150
    talofibular, anatomy 159
    tibio-fibular, rupture, partial 35
      anatomy 159
      sprain 35
    anatomy 159
  calcaneofibular, anatomy 159, 160
    rupture 172
  collateral, hand, anatomy 109
    lateral, anatomy 13, 81
      injury 150
    medial, anatomy 13, 82
      injury 149
      meniscal tear 152
      rupture, complete 35
        partial 35
  coracoacromial, anatomy 64
  cruciate, anatomy 13
    ganglion cyst 153
    injury 151
    MRI 151
  deltoid(ankle), injury 172
  extra-articular, anatomy 13
    injury 35
  hematoma 35
  iliofemoral, anatomy 122, 124, 125
    infant hip 118, 121
  intra-articular 35
  ischiofemoral, anatomy 123
  medial collateral, thumb, anatomy
    109

  peri-articular, anatomy 15
  rupture, complete 35
    healing 35
  sprain 35
  spring, anatomy 178
  talofibular, injury 172
  tibiocalcaneal, anatomy 160, 178
  tibiofibular, anatomy 159
  tibionavicular, anatomy 160
  tibiotalar, anatomy 160
  transverse, anatomy 62
    luxation 73
  triangular carpal, anatomy 13
  ulnar collateral, anatomy 110
lipohemarthrosis 39
lipoma 54
loose bodies 40, 42
  elbow 84
lupus, systemic erythematosus, Achilles
  tendon rupture 165
Lyme disease 41
lymphadenopathy 54
lymphedema 53
lymphoma 53

M

malleolus, fibular, anatomy 159
  lateral, anatomy 159, 160
  medial, anatomy 158, 161, 178
Mallet finger 113
membrane, interosseous, anatomy 155
  compartment syndrome 27
meniscus, see knee
meniscus, lateral, tear 150
  medial, tear 149
  tear 152
    ganglion cyst 153
metacarpal bone, anatomy 107, 110
midfoot, anatomy 176
Milwaukee shoulder 75
Morton, neuroma 187
muscle soleus, posterior tibial tendon
  rupture 170
  abductor, anatomy 122
    brevis, anatomy 124
    digiti, minimi, anatomy 178, 179
    hallucis, anatomy 179
    longus, anatomy 124
    pollicis, anatomy 107
      longus, anatomy 90, 91, 95
  accessory 28
    soleus 173
  adductor, hallucis, anatomy 179
    anatomy 125
    brevis, anatomy 125
    longus, anatomy 125
      rupture 130
    magnus, anatomy 124
      partial tear 130
  anatomy 11
  anterior, tibial, herniation 29
  atrophy 20
    fibrosis 20
    trauma 20
  biceps, anatomy 11, 77, 79, 80
  brachialis, anatomy 77-80, 82
  brachioradialis, anatomy 79-81, 93
  compartment syndrome 26
  contraction 21, 29
  crush injury 23

  delayed-onset soreness 23
  deltoid, anatomy 60-63
    herniation 65
  dorsal, interosseous, anatomy 107,
    109, 177
  elongation 21
  extensor, anatomy 80, 81, 90, 91, 95,
    155
    carpi, radialis, brevis, anatomy 81,
      90, 91
      longus, anatomy 80, 81, 90
    ulnaris, anatomy 91, 95
    digiti minimi, anatomy 91, 95
    digitorum brevis, anatomy 176
    hallucis, brevis, anatomy 176
    indicis, anatomy 91
    pollicis, brevis, anatomy 91
      longus, anatomy 95
  fascia, rupture 29
  fibrosis 27
  flexor, carpi, radialis, anatomy 80
    ulnaris, anatomy 83, 90, 92-94
    digiti minimi, anatomy 178
    digitorum, anatomy 82, 110
      brevis, anatomy 179, 180
        rupture 185
      superficialis, anatomy 80, 91, 93
      longus, anatomy 156
      profundus, anatomy 83, 90, 91,
        93
    hallucis, brevis, anatomy 179
      longus, anatomy 156
    pollicis, longus, anatomy 91
      longus, anatomy 90, 93
  gastrocnemius, anatomy 156, 157
    healing 24
    periosteal desmoid 154
    posterior tibial tendon rupture 170
  gemellus, anatomy 125
  gluteus, maximus, anatomy 123, 125
    calcifications 129
    medius, infant hip, anatomy 121
    minimus, anatomy 122
      infant hip, anatomy 121
  gracilis, pes anserinus tendinitis 147
  hallucis longus, anatomy 155
  healing complications 25
    calcifications 24, 25
    cyst 25
    fibrosis 25
  hematoma 23
  herniation 29
  hypertrophy, exercise 20
  hypothenar, anatomy 107, 110
  iliopsoas, anatomy 122, 124, 125
    anatomy, infant hip 121
    rupture 22
    tendinitis 129
  inferior gemellus, anatomy 123
  infraspinatus, anatomy 63
    glenohumeral joint, effusion 74
  interosseus, anatomy 178, 179
    bursitis 183
    dorsalis, gamekeeper's thumb 116
    palmaris, anatomy 107
    Morton neuroma 187
  lumbricalis, anatomy 107
  myositis ossificans 26
  necrosis 27
  obturator externus, anatomy 124, 125
  ossification 27
  palmaris brevis, anatomy 91, 110

Index

muscle *(cont.)*
  longus, anatomy 90, 91
  pectineus, anatomy 122, 124, 125
  perimysium, anatomy 11
  peroneus brevis, anatomy 155, 156
    longus, anatomy 156, 178
  plantaris, gracilis, anatomy 156
    Achilles tendon rupture 166
  popliteus, anatomy 156
  pronator teres, anatomy 80, 82, 90
  psoas, anatomy, infant hip 118
  quadratus femoris, anatomy 123, 125
    plantaris, anatomy 178–180
  quadriceps, excessive contraction 146
    hematoma 22
    hypertrophy 20
    rupture 146
  rectus femoris, anatomy 124, 125
    infant hip 121
    elongation 21
  rhabdomyolysis 27
  rupture 4,5
    bell-clapper sign 22
    complete 22
    healing 24
    partial 21
    target sign 22
  sartorius, anatomy 122
    anatomy 124, 125
    pes anserinus tendinitis 147
    tendinitis 129
  semimembranosus, accessory 28
  semitendinosus, pes anserinus
    tendinitis 147
  soleus, accessory 28, 173
    rupture 173
    anatomy 156, 157
  supinator, anatomy 79, 90, 91, 95
  thenar, anatomy 107
  tibialis, anterior, anatomy 155
    posterior, anatomy 156
  triceps surae, anatomy 77, 78, 81, 83,
    156
    lipoma 54
  vastus, externus, rupture, partial 24
    intermedius, myositis ossificans 26
      rupture 23
    lateralis, anatomy 122, 125
      infant hip, anatomy 121
      rupture 23
  vastus medialis, foreign body 57

N

needle, *see* puncture
nerve, tibial, anatomy 161
  anatomy 18
    epineurium 18
    fascicles 18
    perineurium 18
  brachial, anatomy 77
  cubital, anatomy 77
  deep peroneal, anatomy 158
  femoral, anatomy 122, 125
    neuritis 45
  inflammation 45
  interdigital, Morton neuroma 187
  median, anatomy 18, 80, 91–93
    carpal canal syndrome 104, 106
    compression 104
  neurinoma 46

neuritis, carpal tunnel syndrome 45
neurofibroma 46
  peroneal, neuritis 45
  plantar digital, Morton neuroma 187
  radial, anatomy 18, 80
  sciatic, anatomy 18, 123
    neurofibroma 46
  ulnar, anatomy 18, 81, 83, 92, 94
    compression 104
    entrapment 88
    Guyon's canal syndrome 104
neuroma, Morton 183, 187

O

olecranon, anatomy 83
  bursitis 85, 89
  entesophyte 87
  fossa, anatomy 82
  loose bodies 84
  tendinitis 87
Osgood-Schlatter disease 145
osteoarthritis, hand 114
osteochondromatosis 41, 75
osteomyelitis, *see* bone

P

pannus 58, 181
patella, luxation 147
  quadriceps tendon, rupture 146
    tendinitis 146
  synovial impingement 147
periosteum, anatomy 14, 26
  metatarsal fracture 184
pes anserinus, comparative study 147
  tendinitis 143, 147
phalanx, anatomy 108, 110
plateau, tibial, fracture 39
plica, synovial 147
process, coracoid, anatomy 64
  coronoid, anatomy 79, 82
  styloid, carpe bossu 99
  ulnar, triangular fibrocartilage tear
    105
prosthesis, abscess 51
  pseudocapsule 51
  silicone 51
pubis, anatomy 124
puncture 58

R

radius, anatomy 79, 90–96
recess, anterior, anatomy, infant hip 18
  suprapatellar, anatomy 41
    anterior, anatomy 158, 159
    effusion 162
    loose body 162
    posterior, anatomy 159
retinaculum, *see* flexor retinaculum and
  synovial impingement
  knee, rupture, acute 147
  medial, synovial impingement 147
  peroneal, luxation 168
rheumatoid arthritis, *see* arthritis
rotator cuff, *see* tendon
runner's knee 150

S

sarcoma, periosteal 26
scaphoid, fracture 99
septum, intermuscular, lateral,
  anatomy 78
  medial, anatomy 78
seronegative spondylarthropathy 165
shin splint, knee 150
shoulder, dislocation 76
  glenoid labrum, joint effusion 74
  impingement syndrome 67, 69, 70
  injury 76
  labrum, posterior, anatomy 16, 63
  myositis ossificans 76
  posterior recess, anatomy 63
skin, anatomy 19
  appendages 19
  cyst 55
  dermis 19
  edema 53
  epidermis, anatomy 19
  Haglund deformity 174
  lipoma 54
  liponecrosis 55
  scar 52
spondylarthropathy, seronegative,
  Achilles tendon rupture 165
  ankle bursitis 171
spondylitis, ankylosing 37
  ankle bursitis 171
sprain, *see* ligament
Stieda-Pellegrini syndrome 149
stress fracture, metarsal bone 184
sustentaculum, tali, anatomy 178
synovitis 39
  pigmented villonodular 41
synovium, anatomy 15
  impingement, knee 147
  profileration, hand 112
  profileration, wrist 103
    rheumatoid arthritis 88
  synovitis, infant hip 127
  thickening, bursitis 37
    hip 126
systemic lupus erythematosus 165

T

talus, anatomy 158, 161, 176
target sign, muscle rupture 22
tendon, tenosynovitis, synovial sheath
  30, 33, 34
  abductor pollicis, De Quervain's
    tenosynovitis 101
    longus, amyloid 106
    anatomy 96
  Achilles, accessory muscle 173
    anatomy 12, 157–159, 161
    cystic mass 175
    Haglund deformity 174
    retrocalcaneal bursitis 171
    rheumatoid arthritis 165
    rupture 9,33, 34, 165, 166
      treatment 166
    tendinitis 163
      acute 7,30, 164
      chronic 31, 163
      nodule 164
      rupture 164
  adductor hallucis, anatomy 179

anatomy 12
anterior tibial, gout 182
  rheumatoid arthritis 181
  tendinitis, chronic 31
biceps femoris, anatomy 123
  anatomy 12, 62
  effusion 70
  impingement syndrome 69
  luxation 73
  rupture 73, 87
    complete 34
    partial 33
  sheath effusion 72
  biceps, tendinitis 72, 87, 143
brachialis, anatomy 79
common, extensor, anatomy 81
  flexor, anatomy 82
empty sheath 34
examination technique 12
extensor, carpi, radialis, brevis,
    anatomy 95, 96
      gout 100
    longus, anatomy 95, 96
  ulnaris, anatomy 94, 96
    rheumatoid arthritis 103
    synovial proliferation 103
digiti minimi, anatomy 96
digitorum and indicis, anatomy 95,
    96
digitorum, longus, anatomy 158,
    177
  anatomy 3,81, 109
  tenosynovitis 102
elbow, anatomy 79
hallucis, longus, anatomy 158, 176
indicis, rupture 113
  tenosynovitis 102
pollicis, brevis, amyloid 106
  anatomy 96
    De Quervain's tenosynovitis
      101
  longus, anatomy 95, 96
    tendinitis, chronic 32
foot, gout 182
flexor, carpi, radialis, anatomy 92, 93
  ulnaris, anatomy 92, 94
    Guyon's canal syndrome 104
  digitorum, anatomy 92, 107, 161
    longus, anatomy 178, 179
    brevis, anatomy 178
    profundus, anatomy 92–94, 108
    superficialis, anatomy 92, 93,
      108
  hallucis, anatomy 178
    longus, anatomy 161, 179
    profundus, anatomy 107
gap 34, 66
hand, rupture 113
  tenosynovitis 111
hip, tendinitis 129
iliopsoas, anatomy 125
infraspinatus, anatomy 60, 61, 64
  calcifications 71
  glenohumeral joint effusion 74
interosseus, anatomy 178
palmaris longus, anatomy 92, 93
  injury 46
patellar, bursitis 148
  jumper's knee 143
  Osgood-Schlatter disease 145
  tendinitis 3, 143, 144
    chronic 31

microrupture 144
  MRI 143
peritendon, anatomy 12
peroneal, ankle bursitis 171
  anatomy 160
  dysplastic 168
  luxation 168
  rupture 168
  tenosynovitis 168
peroneus, brevis, anatomy 160, 177
    planovalgus deformity 170
    tenosynovitis 166
    calcaneal fracture 167
  longus, anatomy 160
pes anserinus, tendinitis 147
plantaris, anatomy 157
  tendinitis 164
popliteal, meniscal tear 152
posterior tibial, rupture 169, 170
  tendinitis, acute 30
  tenosynovitis 169, 175
    MRI 169
  anatomy 161
quadriceps, collection 51
  rupture 146
  tendinitis143, 146
    prepatellar bursitis 148
rectus femoris, anatomy 122, 124
  rupture 130
  tendinitis 129
rotator cuff, absent 75
  anatomy 60, 61
  fibrosis 69
  full thickness tear 65–67
  impingement syndrome 69, 70
  interval, anatomy 62, 64
    bursitis 69
  intrasubstance tear 68
  partial-thickness tear 68
  rupture 67, 69, 71
  tendinitis 32
rupture, complete 33
  partial 33
semimembranosus, anatomy 123
semitendinosus, anatomy 123
sheath, anatomy 12
subscapular, anatomy 63, 64
  calcifications 71
  rupture 73
  tendinitis, chronic 32
supraspinatus, anatomy 60–62
  artifacts 6
  calcifications 71
  full-thickness tear 65
  intrasubstance tear 68
  partial-thickness tear 68
tendinitis, acute 30
  calcification 31, 32, 71, 163
  chronic 31
  knee, chronic, 143
  microruptures 31
tenosynovitis, De Quervain's 101
  hemorrhagic 102
  rheumatoid 102
tibialis, anterior, anatomy 158, 176
  posterior, anatomy 178
triceps, anatomy 82, 83
tennis elbow 86
tensor, fasciae latae, anatomy 122
  infant hip 121
thenar, see eminence and muscle
thrombus, see vein

thumb, anatomy 110
  gamekeeper's 116
  medial collateral ligament, anatomy
    109
  osteoarthritis 114
tibia, anatomy 155, 156, 158, 159
  fracture 48
  shin splint 150
trampoline jumper, shin splint 150
trauma, see injury
triangle, Kager's, anatomy 157, 161
triquetrum, anatomy 94
trochanter, anatomy 123
trochlea, anatomy 79, 80, 82, 83
tuberculosis 41
tuberosity, anterior tibial, bursitis 38
  anterior tibial, fragmentation 145
    Osgood-Schlatter disease 145
  calcaneal, plantar fasciitis 185
tunnel, carpal 104

U

ulna, anatomy 90–96

V

valgus stress, knee 149, 152
varus stress, knee 152
vein, basilar, anatomy 17, 77
  femoral, anatomy 17
  great saphenous, anatomy 158
    thrombus 44
  lateral femoral circumflex, anatomy
    122
  posterior tibial, anatomy 4
  thrombophlebitis 44
  varices 44
vessel, anatomy 14, 17
  anterior tibial, anatomy 155
  brachial, anatomy 77
  Color Doppler 43
  deep femoral, anatomy 125
  foot, anatomy 177
  posterior tibial, anatomy 156, 161
  pseudoaneurysm 43
  superficial femoral, anatomy 125
  talar, anatomy 176

W

wood, see foreign body
wrist, see ganglion cyst and cyst
  arthritis 100
  carpal tunnel syndrome 104
  carpe bossu 99
  gout 100
  Guyon's canal syndrome 104
  rheumatoid arthritis 103
  scaphoid fracture 99
  tenosynovitis 102